American Academy of Pediatrics

A Guide To Starting A Medical Office

Published by:

PUBLISHING
COMPANY

3150 Holcomb Bridge Road, Suite 310, Norcross, GA 30071
770-242-0118

Editor: Kay Stanley
Project Assistant: Bonnie Cole
Art Director: Jeff Weir

Printed in the United States of America

ISBN 0-910761-86-8

American Academy of Pediatrics

Success in pediatrics, whether in an office, hospital, group practice, or staff model health maintenance organization (HMO), depends on mastering basic practice management skills, understanding the many federal and state regulations, and designing strategic plans that can improve the office's performance and profitability. These skills are even more critical if pediatricians are to successfully meet the challenges of managed care. Pediatricians must focus on the key components of practice success: operations, clinical effectiveness, and human resources. Pediatric practices that do this thrive.

To achieve professional success in the practice environment, pediatricians have to form a realistic view of the health care market and create an organization that gives them a competitive advantage in the health care market. The American Academy of Pediatrics Committee on Practice and Ambulatory Medicine (COPAM) recognizes that pediatricians need practical and timely practice management information on topics such as choosing professional advisors, office accounting procedures, leasing space and purchasing equipment, and identifying insurance requirements to assist them in achieving success in practice operations. The manual, *A Guide to Starting a Medical Office,* although written for the general physician community, provides guidance and practical tools on critical practice manage-ment topics also of importance to pediatricians. In addition, the manual includes a variety of checklists, reminders, and sample letters and forms the pediatrician starting in practice, as well as those currently in practice, would find beneficial. Examples include a time line for starting in practice, questionnaires pediatricians can use to evaluate a group practice employment offer, an office supply budget checklist, and medical records checklist.

However, the Committee on Practice and Ambulatory Medicine would like to bring to the reader's attention that some of the information in the manual references Medicare and Workers' Compensation Program policies and procedures. For example, the references to Medicare participation, Medicare Provider Numbers and Medicare Fraud and Abuse regulations are not relevant to pediatricians. Moreover, some of the sample questionnaires and patient surveys are targeted to the patient. These can be revised by the office with minimal effort to refocus them towards the family.

The Committee on Practice and Ambulatory Medicine recommends that you read this manual from cover to cover. It contains a vast amount of critical information pediatricians will need as they begin to decide their initial career choice or are in the midst of changing practice positions. In addition to the practice management techniques and tools referenced in this manual, the Committee would like to point out two valuable practice assessment tools the Academy offers to its members as well as a description of the Academy's managed care resources.

- The Academy's Ambulatory Care Quality Improvement Program (ACQIP) is a complete, results-oriented quality improvement program with an emphasis on self-assessment, peer comparison, and interactive learning. The program is designed to help office-based practitioners to evaluate and improve patient care through continuous quality improvement exercises. ACQIP subscribers have an opportunity to earn four CME Category 1 credits and four risk management credits. If you would like to enroll in the program or have any questions, please call the ACQIP staff at 800-433-9016, ext 4727.

- Another consideration in starting a practice is whether to perform laboratory tests in your office. If you decide to conduct any laboratory tests, you must register with the federal government under the Clinical Laboratory Improvement Amendments (CLIA) of 1988. There are several kinds of laboratory certificates you can obtain, each subject to a varying degree of government regulation. The Academy can orient you on how to set up your laboratory in compliance with CLIA. A major CLIA requirement is proficiency testing for certain regulated tests. The Academy sponsors its own proficiency testing program, AAP-PT, just for pediatric office laboratories. Subscribers to the AAP-PT receive unknown specimens which they test on their in-house equipment and submit answers to the program. Your results are graded and sent back to you and transmitted to the federal Health Care Financing Administration (HCFA) for CLIA compliance. Proficiency testing is an excellent quality improvement tool. It can help you pinpoint the strengths and weaknesses of your laboratory operations. The participant summary reports allow you to compare your laboratory's performance to that of other pediatric office laboratories. For further information on the AAP-PT, contact the Division of Pediatric Practice of the American Academy of Pediatrics at 800-433-9016, ext 7662.

- The Academy's Division of Physician Payment Systems provides tools and information to help pediatricians sort through and adapt to changes taking place in the delivery of medical care. The Division, through its Committees and with input from the Sections, coordinates the Academy's "Strategies for Managed Care Initiative," manages the pediatric RBRVS project, responds to member queries on CPT and ICD-9-CM coding, creates practice management informational resources, and develops policy on child health financing and delivery issues. The Committee on Child Health Financing, a constituent Committee of the Division, developed the manual *A Pediatrician's Guide to Managed Care.* With over 200 pages of information, the guide supplies critical advice pediatricians can use immediately for negotiating contracts, evaluating capitation rates, assessing physician organization models, and clarifying legal issues. For information on ordering this manual, contact the Academy's Division of Marketing and Publications at 800/433-9016. For information on the Division of Physician Payment Systems and its activities, please call the staff at 800-433-9016, ext 7917.

The American Academy of Pediatrics is committed to the attainment of optimal physical, mental, and social health for all infants, children, adolescents, and young adults. To this end, the members of the Academy dedicate their efforts and resources. The Academy welcomes members in eleven categories: Fellow, Specialty Fellow, Candidate Fellow, Post-Residency Training Fellow, Resident Fellow, Honoree Fellow, Emeritus Fellow, Subscriber Fellow, Subscriber Affiliate, Corresponding Fellow, and Canadian Paediatric Society/AAP Dual Fellow. For further information about requirements and benefits of AAP membership or for membership application materials, contact the Division of Member Services at 800-433-9016, ext 7386, 4720, or 7863.

About The Coker Group

Since 1987, The Coker Group has earned a national reputation for helping providers succeed in the wake of reform, grow in a potentially troublesome environment, and to continue to deliver quality, cost-effective health care to their communities. We specialize in assisting our clients in these areas:

Programs and Services:

- Physician Network Development
- Practice Assessments
- Practice Valuations and Acquisition Negotiations
- Practice Brokerage Services
- Physician Employment and Compensation Contract Design
- Group Practice Development
- Practice Management Services
- Management Services Organization (MSO) Development
- Practice Start-up
- Educational Programs
- Evaluation and Consultant Services

For more information, contact:

THE
Coker
GROUP
National Consultants to Healthcare Providers

The Coker Group / 3150 Holcomb Bridge Road / Suite 310
Norcross, Georgia 30071 / 770-242-0118

About The Book

A Guide to Starting a Medical Office addresses the nuts and bolts of establishing a medical practice as a business in the world of managed care. While there is much to learn, there has likely been little to prepare you for this part of your experience. The following questions are but a few of those that will arise as you enter practice.

- What corporate structure is best?

- Where should the practice be located?

- What equipment is needed?

- Where do you purchase equipment?

- What medical and business supplies are needed?

- How much will this cost?

- Where do I begin?

The nature of medical practice is constantly changing—and will be in the foreseeable future. This book provides guidelines on the aspects of business to consider when entering practice. It will guide you in critical decisions involving location and type of practice versus practicing as an employee of a medical institution. It will provide valuable advice on the handling of personnel, patients and accounts.

What information can the reader find?

The reader will find practical and specific information for use in the day-to-day operation of the medical practice, including:

- How to determine an area's need for a physician

- A time line for starting to practice medicine

- Guidelines for assessing the type of medical practice that is right for you

- Tax and licensing requirements

- Office accounting procedures

- Managing personnel

- Keeping proper medical records

- Developing policies and procedures

- Billing and collections

- Risk management

- Marketing strategies

A Guide to Starting a Medical Office is based on up-to-date techniques in practice management. As publishers, we are committed to providing the most current information concerning topics of interest for the "business side of medicine." For more information on resources available, contact us at the following address:

Coker Publishing, LLC
3150 Holcomb Bridge Road
Suite 310
Norcross, GA 30071
770-242-0118
800-345-5829

Editor
Kay Stanley

Overview

Whether you are establishing a solo practice or joining a group, beginning the practice of medicine requires considerable forethought. The process should begin—at a minimum—one year before your transition into private practice. With careful consideration and planning, your pathway will be much smoother and less stressful.

Generally, time lines serve as effective road maps for project management. The purpose of this book is to set forth a well-planned time line for starting your practice. By following these guidelines, you will move efficiently through the maze of procedures for acquiring licensing and insurance, and for meeting the other requirements for medical practice.

This book is essential for every physician who is entering practice for the first time. It will help you understand the "business-side" of medical practice by providing sensible information applicable to the practice of medicine. Some topics are:

- the art of managing people

- the implementation of sound financial procedures

- guarding against malpractice and other risk management considerations, and

- compliance with regulations and statutes.

Completing every task included in the time line may not be necessary for you. For instance, if you are joining an established partnership or group, you likely will not be leasing office space or purchasing equipment. However, as your practice grows, expands or relocates, this information will serve as good advice. The principles presented are timeless and applicable to virtually every practice, whatever the locale.

Now that we have set the stage, let's get started!

Table of Contents

CHAPTER 1

Selecting a Practice Location

Factors Influencing Your Decision

One of the most important decisions you will make as a new physician is where you will practice. This decision may hinge on the opportunities you have been offered, or the opportunities you seek may be based on your geographic preferences.

Before you begin to research a geographic location, think about what your ideal location would be, where you would be the happiest, and what you want to get out of the practice of medicine. Will you start a private practice, join a group or seek employment with a hospital or other entity? Considerations might include prospects for your continued development as a physician, likelihood of financial success, and whether the needs of your family, including professional opportunities for your spouse and good schools for your children, can be met.

Several major factors will influence your choice of practice location:

Professional Relationships and Opportunities. These include the relationships you have formed during medical school and with practicing physicians who have influenced your career. Professional opportunities encompass what an area offers for continuing education, professional stimulation, and the opportunity to practice in a hospital offering the most advanced technology and facilities. You will want to consider whether the area provides opportunities for professional growth for your spouse.

Prior Exposure. Where you went to medical school, your residency program, and your place of birth may all influence your choice of location. Nearly 50 percent of physicians who practice in towns with populations less than 2,500 grew up in towns of similar size. Studies suggest that there is also a strong relationship between location of postgraduate training and location of private practice.

Economic Factors. Salary or income potential and cost of living are also strong determinants in the choice of geographic location. You will want to know if the location you choose is in an area of need, in a depressed economy, or in an area of rapid growth. Depending on your specialty, you should learn whether the growth in the area is due to an influx of young families or is the result of a booming retirement community.

Small towns where the community is medically under served often provide opportunities for the highest income. Research the demographics of the location you choose for population, the per capita income, age and gender mix.

Environmental Factors. Quality and availability of housing, cultural opportunities, and the educational system should all be considered in your selection. Proximity to a major airport, public transportation and recreational opportunities will influence your decision. Finally, climate and even pollution may be factors to consider.

Other Determinants. Hospital proximity, religious affiliations, group practice opportunities, and the availability of other physicians with whom you might share call are important. The new physician entering solo practice will also want to check availability and average cost per square foot for office space.

Take the time to write down your objectives, constraints, assumptions, and goals for success. Use your goals and objectives to help you in the decision-making process. Many sources are available for obtaining information about practice opportunities in geographic locations that best suit your needs.

Where to Look for Employment Opportunities

- MD Direct (see Chapter 3 for more information)
- Residency Program Directors
- American Medical Association's placement service
- Specialty Society placement service
- State and County medical societies
- Classified ads in journals (e.g., *Journal of The American Medical Association, New England Journal of Medicine,* and specialty journals).

Where to Find Information Concerning a Geographic Location

- Regional Planning Commission
- Census Bureau (local offices are available in major cities and state capitals). You must be specific about the information you need.
- State Department of Tourism
- Area Chamber of Commerce
- Local and State Medical Societies

How to Determine the Area's Need for a Physician

- County or State Medical Society
- Chief of Staff at the area hospital(s)
- Other physicians
- Pharmacists
- Local Health Systems Agency (if available) can provide critical information about physician demographics, hospital beds, occupancy rates, under served areas and other health care delivery systems such as ambulatory care centers, family planning clinics, and physician extenders.

- Sunday newspapers from the areas you are considering. You may wish to subscribe or arrange to purchase these.

Once you have narrowed your options to two or three locations, visit these areas at least once before making a final selection. Visit the local hospitals and talk with the Chiefs of Staff. Determine how long it will take you to obtain hospital privileges. Make sure the hospital(s) is not closed to new staff members.

If you are planning to open a practice of your own, you will need at least twelve (12) months lead time to do your research, select a location, and complete other necessary arrangements. Since so many details are involved, we have provided a time line for you. Using this will insure your awareness of everything that you must accomplish before joining a group or opening your own practice and within the specified time.

You can delegate some objectives on the timetable to your spouse or other individual that you trust. That person will need to be persistent and pay attention to detail. You, the physician, should take the responsibility of seeing that all the requirements are completed on time.

You will be asked to provide copies of all your licenses, identifier numbers, and other credentialing requirements several times. To prepare, begin now to build a file that includes the original and several copies of this information to provide as needed.

Time Line for Starting to Practice Medicine

Photocopy this time line and keep it with you. Work on completing these steps whenever you have a moment to devote.

Not all requirements will apply to all practice options. We have coded each line:

E   for an employed physician
GP   for physicians joining a group practice
SP   for the physician starting a solo private practice.

One Year Before Starting Practice

		Check off as completed:	Responsible Party:
1.	Make final decision on practice location. (E, GP, SP)	❑	_____
2.	Check on membership for: (E, GP, SP)		
	County medical society	❑	_____
	State medical society	❑	_____
	American Medical Association	❑	_____
	Specialty society	❑	_____
3.	For comparison purposes, get in writing details of contracts from groups or corporations you are considering joining. (GP, E) (See group practice questionnaire in Chapter 3.)	❑	_____
4.	Begin to examine net worth in terms of capital available for start-up costs. (SP) (See Chapter 9.)	❑	_____
5.	If possible, reserve office phone number, (or answering service number). (SP)	❑	_____
6.	Find out the date when telephone books are printed. Have your name listed in both the white and yellow pages. (SP)	❑	_____
7.	Visit banks and begin shopping for a loan. Pick up loan applications and meet loan officers. Determine what information the bank needs to evaluate your loan application. (SP) (See Chapter 9.)	❑	_____
8.	Open:		
	Checking account, personal. (E, GP, SP)	❑	_____
	Checking account, business. (SP)	❑	_____
	Savings account, personal. (E, GP, SP)	❑	_____
	Savings account, business. (SP)	❑	_____

9. Draw up an income/expenditure projection for
    first year of practice. Talk with several bankers
    regarding borrowing money; submit applications.
    (SP) (See Chapter 9, Developing a Business Plan.)   ❑   _____

Nine Months Before Starting Practice

1. Check sites for leasing/buying medical office
    space. (SP)   ❑   _____

2. Check zoning ordinances with your local city
    hall and/or zoning board regarding signage,
    type of businesses allowed in the area; ask about
    any anticipated changes. (SP)   ❑   _____

3. Check on utility requirements for the office. (SP)   ❑   _____

4. If leasing, see if any leasehold improvements
    are needed and when you can start making these
    improvements. (SP) (See Chapter 10.)   ❑   _____

5. Determine office layout and design. (SP)   ❑   _____

6. Determine office and medical equipment needed.
    If installing x-ray equipment, check with the state
    health department, radiological health section, to see
    if they require special registration or certificate. Make
    the same checks for laboratory or outpatient surgery
    facilities. (SP) (See Chapter 4 for laboratory license
    information.)   ❑   _____

7. Choose advisors (as appropriate). (See Chapter 7.)

        Accountant (E, GP, SP)   ❑   _____

        Attorney (E, GP, SP)   ❑   _____

        Banker (E, GP, SP)   ❑   _____

        Insurance broker(s) (E, GP, SP)   ❑   _____

        Management consultant (SP)   ❑   _____

        Real estate broker (E, GP, SP)   ❑   _____

        Other (e.g., computer consultant)   ❑   _____

8. Evaluate office lease and/or partnership agreement
    contracts with your attorney before you sign them.
    (See Chapters 3 and 10.)   ❑   _____

9. Obtain bids on major office equipment you will need;
    compare leasing versus purchasing. Be sure to get a
    written guarantee of delivery date and in-transit insurance.
    (See equipment list and budget in Chapter 10.)

        Dictation equipment (SP)   ❑   _____

Intercom system (determine whether you want it separate from telephones) (SP) ❏ _____

Exam room/medical equipment (SP) ❏ _____

Photocopy machine (SP) ❏ _____

Computer/typewriter/word processor (SP) ❏ _____

Telephone equipment (SP) ❏ _____

Calculator (SP) ❏ _____

Light signaling system (SP) ❏ _____

Reception room/office furniture and decorations (SP) ❏ _____

Tool kit/flashlight (SP) ❏ _____

10. If in a partnership, complete the details of the partnership agreement; have it drawn up and signed by each partner.

11. Obtain narcotics license: (E, GP, SP)

Federal: Application for registration available through the Department of Justice, Drug Enforcement Administration, local or state office. If necessary, contact the national office: Drug Enforcement Administration, P.O. Box 28083, Central Station, Washington, D.C., 20005, 202 724 1013. ❏ _____

State: Check with your local medical licensing board to see who issues licenses in your state. The state pharmacy board or the Department of Registration and Education usually does this. ❏ _____

12. Inform the state medical licensing board of your new address. (E, GP, SP) ❏ _____

Six Months Before Starting Practice

1. Obtain the services of an answering service: (SP)

Physicians' exchange (hospital or medical society) (E, SP, GP) ❏ _____

Personal (office) (SP) ❏ _____

Beeper service (SP) ❏ _____

Call forwarding (SP) ❏ _____

2. Select a Pension Plan or Individual Retirement Account. (SP) ❏ _____

3. Check with the medical society regarding their position and guidelines on advertising in the local newspaper, and other forms of announcements. Many will provide mailing labels and assist with printing. (SP) ❏ _____

4. Meet with the professional representative from the Medicare fiscal intermediary (the local medical society will advise you which company this is), Medicaid (administered by your state health and human services agency), and major commercial carriers regarding: (See Chapter Four.) ❏ _____

   Provider number(s) (SP, E, GP, check with employer) ❏ _____

   Medicare fee schedule (SP) ❏ _____

5. Obtain a current procedural terminology book (CPT-4). (SP) ❏ _____

6. Obtain an International Classification of Diseases Book (ICD-9-CM). (SP) ❏ _____

7. Apply for hospital staff privileges. (SP, E, GP) ❏ _____

8. Arrange to attend Grand Rounds at the local hospital(s). (SP, E, GP) ❏ _____

9. Order medical record system. (SP)

10. Order sign for office. (SP)

11. Obtain insurance forms (HCFA 1500 Claim Form from the AMA: 800 621 8335).

12. Notify pharmaceutical representatives and other appropriate sales persons that you are setting up practice. ❏ _____

13. Obtain county and city occupational licenses available from the county/city clerk's office or city hall. (See Chapter 4.) ❏ _____

Three Months Before Starting Practice

1. Arrange for professional malpractice insurance. (SP, GP, E; check with employer) ❏ _____

2. Arrange for office insurance (Call 800 458 5736 for information on AMA-sponsored insurance plan. (SP) (See Chapter 8.)

   Office overhead (SP) ❏ _____

   Office liability (SP) ❏ _____

Business interruption (SP) ❏ _____

Employee fidelity bond (SP) ❏ _____

Office contents (SP)

Umbrella: Provides comprehensive catastrophic liability coverage for liability claims beyond the limits of your regular liability programs. (SP) ❏ _____

Workers' Compensation: This is often required by law and is determined on a state-by-state basis. Check with your state's workers' compensation board or industrial commission. (SP) ❏ _____

Health: Major medical for yourself, dependents and employees. ❏ _____

Disability (SP, E, GP; check with employer) ❏ _____

Life (SP, E, GP) ❏ _____

Automobile (SP, E, GP) ❏ _____

3. Arrange for telephone service installation. Consider purchasing telephone equipment. (SP) ❏ _____

4. Consider a money market fund, opened directly or with your bank. (SP) ❏ _____

5. Consider arranging for acceptance of credit cards (VISA, MasterCard, American Express, etc.) in your office through your local bank. (Call 800 366 6968 for information on the AMA-sponsored VISA program.) (SP) ❏ _____

6. Talk with the local newspaper regarding practice announcement ads.

7. Order office opening announcements. (SP) ❏ _____

8. Arrange to give talks to community groups on health topics. (SP, GP) (See Chapter 15.) ❏ _____

9. Meet physicians who are potential referral sources. Send letters, arrange appointments. (SP, GP) ❏ _____

10. Find out if a patient referral service is available through the local medical society. Send them essential information. (SP, GP) ❏ _____

11. Check on memberships in civic and church organizations. (SP, E, GP) ❏ _____

12. Arrange for movers, if necessary. (SP, E, GP) ❏ _____

13. Write to your State Department of Labor for state employment regulations and Wage and Hour information. (SP) ❏ _____

14. Write preliminary job descriptions for employees. (SP) ❏ _____

15. Write policy manual for your office employees. (SP) ❏ _____

16. Check local resources for personnel. (SP) ❏ _____

17. Start interviewing for office/clinical personnel. (SP) ❏ _____

18. Apply for your Federal Employer Identification Number through your local Internal Revenue Service Office, (SS-4 Form). (SP) ❏ _____

19. Apply for your State Employer Identification Number through your state employment office/labor department. (SP) ❏ _____

20. Obtain "Small Business Tax Guide" and your Federal Estimated Income Tax Form through your local IRS office, or attend Small Business Tax Seminar at your local IRS office. (SP) ❏ _____

21. Write for your State Estimated Income Tax Form through your state employment office/labor department. (SP) ❏ _____

22. Obtain payroll withholding booklets (federal, state, city) through your local IRS office. (SP) ❏ _____

23. Review tax requirements with your accountant. (SP) ❏ _____

24. Plan and order appointment scheduling book. (SP) ❏ _____

25. Arrange for, as needed:

    Janitorial service ❏ _____

    Snow removal ❏ _____

    Laundry service ❏ _____

    Grounds maintenance ❏ _____

26. Order clinical supplies and set up inventory control system. (SP) (See Chapter 10.) ❏ _____

27. Order business supplies: (SP)

    Appointment cards ❏ _____

    Business cards ❏ _____

    Patient recall system ❏ _____

    Petty cash vouchers ❏ _____

    Letterhead stationery and envelopes ❏ _____

    Stationery supplies (e.g., postage scale, meter) ❏ _____

    Deposit stamp for checks ❏ _____

    Prescription pads ❏ _____

    Purchase order forms ❏ _____

Preprinted telephone message pads ❑ _____

28. Determine likely office hours based on community need. (SP) ❑ _____

29. Determine fee schedule. (SP) ❑ _____

30. Select and order magazines: (SP)

For reception room ❑ _____

Medical journals for yourself ❑ _____

31. Purchase office equipment and furniture; arrange delivery date. (SP)

32. Arrange for: (SP)

Laboratory services for your patients ❑ _____

X-ray services for your patients ❑ _____

33. Notify area pharmacies that you are starting practice. (GP, SP) ❑ _____

34. Write patient information booklet and have it printed. (SP) ❑ _____

One Month Before Starting Practice

1. Start setting up office. (SP) ❑ _____

2. Have utilities turned on:

Telephone ❑ _____

Electricity ❑ _____

Gas ❑ _____

Water ❑ _____

3. Start accepting appointments. (SP) ❑ _____

4. Hire and train office personnel regarding: (SP)

Telephone techniques ❑ _____

Collections ❑ _____

Appointments ❑ _____

Office policies ❑ _____

5. Decide on collection/insurance policy. (SP) ❑ _____

6. Hang out shingle (post sign). (SP) ❑ _____

7. Establish a petty cash fund. (SP) ❑ _____

8. Establish a change fund. (SP) ❑ _____

9. Place announcement in community paper and
   medical society bulletin: (SP, GP)

   Advertisement ❏ _____

   News release ❏ _____

10. Mail out announcements to physicians, pharmacists,
    hospitals, health groups. (SP, GP) ❏ _____

11. Plan office "open house." (SP)

Opening Day of Office

1. See first patient. ❏ _____

2. Congratulate yourself. You are now in practice! ❏ _____

CHAPTER 2

Choosing a Corporate Structure

Types of Medical Practices

Under existing laws, there are four major kinds of medical practices that can be established.

- Solo (can also be incorporated)
- Partnerships (two or more physicians)
- Corporations (one or more physicians)
- Limited Liability Corporation (one or more physicians)

Group practices can have several variations, including nonprofit practices, foundations, and associations, in addition to the more typical partnerships and corporate practices.

Solo Practice

The major reason a physician chooses solo practice is to maintain autonomy. Solo practice allows the physician to "rule the roost," so to speak, and to establish the practice guidelines, office hours, policies and procedures that he or she prefers.

This type of practice can be either a sole proprietorship or a professional corporation. In a sole proprietorship, the physician is personally liable for all the debt and legal infractions of the practice. The tax status is simplified in that the physician uses a Schedule C (profit and loss from business) form to file for his practice earnings and expenses.

Tax consequences: self employment tax; Medicare—2.9 percent. (Count on one-third of every net dollar as tax).

Partnership

A partnership is "an association of two or more persons for the purpose of carrying on as co-owners of a business for profit." Partners invest in their business to make a profit.

The advantages of a partnership are:

- Each partner has equal rights in the management and conduct of the partnership.
- No one can become a partner without the consent of all the other partners.
- Partners have the right to a formal accounting of partnership affairs.
- Each partner has the responsibility to sustain a fiduciary relationship with the other partners.
- Financial and professional risks and responsibilities are shared.

Disadvantages:

- All partners are liable for each individual partner's wrong acts under the partnership.

- Individual partners also are liable for acts of commission or omission assumed by the partnership as a whole.

- Partnership losses must be divided equally among the partners or based on some prearranged schedule.

- The partnership can neither sue nor be sued per se; however, individual partners are liable for any suit against a partner if the suit concerns the principal nature of the business, in this case medicine.

Corporate Practice

Corporate practice reduces the personal and financial risk to the individual physician, while also providing opportunities to shelter income through a qualified retirement program.

Advantages to Incorporation:

- There is limited liability to the individual physician.

- There is centralized management, with a formal organization in which authority and responsibility are assigned to appropriate parties.

- Continuity of life means the corporation will last beyond the careers of the present physicians.

- Ownership interest can be transferred easily through the sale of stock representing the value of the corporation's assets.

- Pension and profit-sharing plans are superior to those available in a partnership.

- The arrangement can save on taxes.

- The corporation can pay for medical and hospital insurance benefits, a $50,000 life insurance plan, a disability program, (making it an expense to the corporation and therefore tax deductible).

Disadvantages of a Corporation:

- Only physicians can be shareholders.

- Double taxation is imposed on the physicians' salaries and on the profits of the corporation. Seeing that the corporation has few, if any, profits can offset this.

- Corporations cost money to establish and initiate costly legal fees and higher Social Security payments for the physicians. (Attorneys' fees run approximately $250 plus per hour.)

- Managing a corporation requires extensive organization, e.g., board meetings with accurate minutes, formal notices of annual and quarterly meetings, election of officers, and proper revision of bylaws and articles of incorporation, as required.

- A biannual registration fee of $150 to medical licensing board is required.

Tax Consequences: taxed on personal salary and corporate profits; separate tax return

Limited Liability Corporation

A fourth option, the limited liability corporation or LLC, has recently been recognized by the IRS as an approved corporate structure. It provides the owners with the best advantages of both the corporation and the partnership. An LLC is not legal in every state. Check with your attorney or legal department to verify that your state recognizes the LLC as a legal corporation. While the LLC structure is appropriate for most forms of business, state law in some states sets up a parallel structure for doctors, lawyers, accountants and other professionals called a Professional LLC.

Under Professional LLC provisions, members are not liable for the overall obligations of the LLC; however, each member is liable for any negligence, wrongful act or misconduct committed by him or by any person under his direct supervision while rendering services on behalf of the LLC.

Membership in the Professional LLC may only be transferred to other professionals who are eligible. At least one of the professionals forming an LLC must be authorized (licensed) to render professional services in the state where the LLC is formed. In the case of a medical LLC, all members must be licensed in that state.

Advantages:

- The personal liability of each member of an LLC is limited to his personal investment in the LLC. This means that no member of the LLC is personally liable for the debts of the entire organization.

- The LLC offers pass-through tax benefits; that is, there is no entity-level tax on the entity's income, but only a tax on the individual's share of the entity's income.

Other Features:

- *Ownership.* An LLC is owned by its members. To ensure pass-through tax benefits, membership in the LLC may not be transferred without consent of a majority of the LLC's members. Anyone can be an LLC member.

- The LLC may be managed by its members or by one or more managers appointed by the members.

- LLC members generally vote in proportion to their ownership interests, and all matters require the approval of a majority of the members.

- As with any other type of business, the LLC must obtain a certificate of authority to do business in another state. However, the other state must recognize the LLC structure and its qualification requirements.

Office-Sharing Arrangements

While this not a legal structure, some physicians choose this arrangement to share the cost of operations with another physician. The two parties should maintain a written agreement concerning their arrangement.

Patients should be aware that the two physicians have separate practices. If there is no written agreement, and patients assume that the physicians are "partners," both physicians may be implicated in a malpractice litigation.

The written agreement should include the following.

- A statement of purpose. Example:
  "This agreement is solely for the purpose of sharing office space for the practice of medicine and is not an agreement creating a partnership between the two parties."

- Names of the parties involved, the location of the office, whether both parties enter into the lease, or one physician sublets or leases a part of his owned space to another physician; the term of the lease agreement.

- How the office space will be allocated.

- How expenses will be allocated, i.e., equally, based on allocated space, by predetermined formula, or borne separately.

- Allocation of personnel. Sharing employees carries some risks for the physicians. It is recommended that each physician employ his/her own employees.

- Provisions for purchase of equipment and furniture.

- General liability insurance/health insurance coverage. This may be purchased as one policy at considerable savings to both physicians. Check with your insurance agent.

- Provisions in case of death of one of the physicians

- Provisions if one physician wishes to end the agreement, e.g., assignment of telephone number, division of furniture and equipment, substitution of another tenant, etc.

CHAPTER 3

Considering Employment Options

Assessing Group Practice and Employment Opportunities

According to the American Medical Association Health Policy Research Center, the proportion of self-employed physicians dropped from 68.1 percent in 1990 to 39.4 percent in 1995. Solo practice is not as favored today because of the expense of operations, excessive paperwork, increasing rules and regulations, and the problems of managing employees each day. Although solo physicians have difficulty in negotiating favorable managed care contracts, solo practices remain popular in rural areas where managed care is not an influential factor.

As stated previously, the predominant reason a physician chooses solo practice is to have autonomy, the freedom to establish the practice guidelines, office hours, policies and procedures that he or she prefers. Solo practice permits the flexibility and personal attention to patients that group practices often forfeit.

The insurgence of managed care has caused an increase in the number of physicians joining group practices or seeking employment with a hospital or Health Maintenance Organization. Most group practices bring new physicians in under an employment contract. After a designated period, they may offer the employed physician an opportunity to buy into the practice. Other groups will allow new physicians to buy in immediately.

The purpose of this chapter is to give you information that will allow you to make an informed decision about joining a group practice. Topics included are the advantages and disadvantages of joining a group, what to look for in a contract, and how to evaluate the character and effectiveness of a group. This chapter will also help you if you wish to investigate employment opportunities with hospitals and HMOs and incorporates tips on what to look for in an employment contract.

Advantages of Group Practice

- Fewer problems establishing office operations and building a patient load.
- Less initial financing needed.
- Less financial risk involved, providing greater initial security.
- Regular work schedules, yielding more time for family/personal pursuits.
- Shared coverage for night call, weekends, and holidays.
- Coverage for vacations, sick days, and continuing education.
- Professional atmosphere and shared knowledge afforded by group relationships.
- Greater access to technology and trained personnel.

- Increased opportunities to pursue research and/or administrative interests.
- Fewer problems involved in retirement or decreased work load.
- Greater competitive advantages because of a larger market share.

Disadvantages of Group Practice

- Loss of autonomy; decisions made by consensus.
- Greater potential for conflicts with associates over personal differences, income distribution, group expenditures and investments, group procedures, and policies and philosophies on patient care.
- Pressure to refer patients to physicians within the group (especially in a multi specialty group).
- Greater likelihood of impersonality in dealing with patients.
- Possible liability for any errors made by associates or losses incurred by the group.
- Greater difficulty in effecting change.
- Uneven distribution of cases.

Where to Obtain Information on Group Practice and Partnership Opportunities

- Residency programs
- Medical schools
- Specialty society placement service
- State, county and local medical societies
- Physician recruiting firms
- Classified ads in journals and metropolitan newspapers
- Hospital administrators or hospital marketing departments
- Chiefs of staff
- Multi site clinic and hospital management firms
- Preferred Provider Organizations (PPOs)
- Health Maintenance Organizations (all types)
- Personal contacts including pharmaceutical representatives and durable medical equipment representatives
- Established group practices
- American Group Practice Association, Placement Services
- Practice brokers
- Management consultants
- MD Direct
  3150 Holcomb Bridge Road, Suite 205
  Norcross, GA 30071
  888 MD DIRECT; 888 633 4732

An online service with a membership of more than 100,000 physicians, MD Direct has search and research capabilities. This service provides hospitals, group practices, and managed care organizations with information about available physicians who fit specific criteria. This online service gives physicians dozens of employment opportunities (both permanent and Locum Tenens) in many geographic locations.

- Group Practice Associations:

American Group Practice Association
1422 Duke Street
Alexandria, VA 22314
703 838 0033

Medical Group Management Association
104 Inverness Terrace East
Englewood, CO 80112-5306
303 799 1111

Signing an Employment Contract

Before signing any type of employment agreement, you need to know what to look for and how to interpret the contract language. It is also important to understand that you have some room for negotiation. After reading the contract, define any points that cause you concern. Rank these concerns in order of importance. Negotiate firmly on the most important issues and be willing to concede in areas of less interest.

Employment contracts generally include the following clauses:

The Term of the Contract

- Does the contract become effective on the date it is signed or on the day you start to work?

- Length of the contract

- Does it have an automatic renewal? Is it subject to renegotiation at the time of renewal?

Duties

- What hours is the employee expected to work and what specific call duties will the employee be expected to handle?

- Is the employee restricted in any way from seeking additional employment outside of the practice?

- What kinds of patients will be assigned to the employed physician?

- What restrictions does the physician employee have regarding the acceptance of patients and modes of treatment?

- What penalties, if any, are incurred if the employee voluntarily terminates employment before the contract expires?

- What provisions will apply if the employee is called to jury duty? To military duty?

Compensation

- What salary will the employee receive?

- How will the salary be computed?

- At what intervals and increments will the salary increase?

- What incentive bonuses apply and how are they calculated?

Benefits

- Are pension and profit-sharing plans available? What is the vesting schedule?

- Will the employer pay the employee's malpractice insurance premiums?

- Who pays for "tail" insurance? (See Chapter 8 for discussion of "tail" insurance.)

- Will the physician employees participate in the group life insurance plan?

- What additional fringe benefits will the employee receive?
  - Vacation
  - Sick leave/discretionary days
  - CME/conventions/postgraduate work
  - Professional books and periodicals
  - Professional dues
  - Medical equipment
  - Office space
  - Clerical help
  - Automobile allowance
  - Moving allowance

Buy-In Agreement

- On what date will the employee be allowed to acquire part ownership in the practice? What percentage of the practice will the employee be able to purchase at buy-in?

- What will part ownership in the practice entail? Specifically, what percentage of the following will be owned by the new partner?
  - Accounts receivable
  - Equipment
  - Goodwill
  - Supply inventory and prepaid items
  - Office buildings and real estate location
  - Liabilities

- What will be the cost to the employee to buy into the practice?

- How will the value of the practice be determined?

- What are the exact terms of payment of the buy-in?
  - Lump payments or extended payments
  - Rate of interest

Covenant Not to Compete (Restrictive Covenant)

- Will the employee be asked to sign a covenant not to compete? What are the specific terms of such a covenant?

- How enforceable is a covenant not to compete in the state where signed?

- Is there a time limit beyond which a signed covenant not to compete no longer applies?

- Are there any other clauses in this contract that impose certain obligations or restrictions on the employee?

- Will the employed physician be allowed a trial period before agreeing to a restrictive covenant?

Termination

- Can either the physician or employer terminate the contract with 30 days notice?

- Does the contract terminate on death of the employee, or will the employee's family or estate be subject to contractual obligations?

- Under which, if any, of the following conditions will the contract automatically terminate?
  - Loss of hospital privileges
  - Suspension, revocation or cancellation of employee's right to practice medicine
  - Employee refuses to follow practice policies or procedures
  - Employee commits an act of gross negligence
  - Employee is convicted of a crime
  - Employee becomes impaired due to alcohol or drug abuse
  - Breach of contract terms
  - Employee becomes disabled (How many days, etc.?)

Understanding Restrictive Covenants

A restrictive covenant, or a covenant not to compete, may be defined as follows:

> "An express provision of an employment contract or a partnership agreement that restricts the right of the employee or associate, after the conclusion of his or her term of employment, to engage in a business similar to or competitive with that of the employer, partner, or seller of the practice."

Such restrictions, usually, are limited to a specified time and geographical area. In jurisdictions in which there are no statutory limitations on restrictive covenants, the general rule is that the courts will enforce such covenants if they are "reasonable" in view of all of the circumstances of a particular case. In assessing the reasonableness of a particular restrictive covenant, a court will consider three major tests of "reasonableness," as follows:

- The covenant is no greater than necessary to protect the employer in some legitimate interest.

- It is not unduly harsh and oppressive on the employee.

- It is not injurious to the public interest.

Each case is decided individually; differing time limits and geographical restrictions could be judged reasonable in a particular case. Courts tend to enforce restrictive covenants in contracts more often for the sale of a practice or business than in employment or partnership contracts.

A physician contemplating employment should not sign a contract containing a restrictive covenant without obtaining legal advice. If the employer insists on a covenant, the physician may wish to negotiate the following:

- A trial period before the restrictive covenant becomes operative;

- An eventual limitation after which the covenant is no longer in force

- A provision that states that the restrictive covenant is null and void if the employee is discharged without adequate reason, or if the employee leaves for just cause.

Income Distribution and Expense Allocation

Some groups pay each physician a salary and a portion of net revenues, if any, that remain after paying expenses and physician salaries. This excess may be paid to each physician equally or distributed according to a formula. If you will be receiving a base salary and participating in the distribution of net revenues, be sure you understand how it is calculated.

Methods of Income Distribution

Following are various examples of income distribution that you may encounter in practice options:

Equal Distribution. Each member receives an equal share of the practice revenue.

Productivity. Members are compensated based on the amount they generate in individual patient charges.

Formulas. Several factors, weighed by importance, are used to determine remuneration. Some of these factors are as follows:

- Goodwill/longevity
- Stock ownership
- Productivity
- Board Certification
- Administrative roles (managing partner, etc.)
- New patients
- Referral sources
- Teaching/faculty position

Each factor in the formula is given percentage points. Physicians in the group must decide how many points will be given to each factor. If points are allocated for longevity, there should be a maximum that each doctor can earn.

Note: The Stark II legislation now prevents groups from compensating a physician based on how much revenue that physician generates for ancillary services such as lab and x-ray. However, revenues from ancillary services may be distributed equally to each physician in the group, regardless of whether he generated these revenues.

Methods of Expense Allocation

Equal assessments. This is the easiest method. The expenses are subtracted from the gross revenue, and the net income is available for physician distribution.

Direct costs. Any costs incurred for the benefit of a physician are charged directly to that physician. This allows each physician to have any equipment or personnel that he prefers.

Indirect costs. Costs such as rent, utilities, and maintenance are charged to each physician, usually as a per-square-foot charge. This way, each physician pays only for what he or she uses.

Expenses as a percentage of productivity. Each physician is charged for expenses at the same rate he generates income for the group. If the physician generates 40 percent of the income, he is charged 40 percent of the expenses. In a multi specialty group, the surgical specialists may object to this type of allocation because primary care physicians typically use much more space than other physicians.

	Positives	Negatives
Solo Practice	■ Independence ■ Clinical autonomy ■ Immediate rewards for efficiency	■ Risk for practice and clinical management ■ Must develop own patient base ■ No financial cushion
Small Independent Group Practice	■ Greater role in governance than in larger group ■ Shared risk and overhead	■ Responsible for colleagues' performance ■ Less independence than solo ■ Shared financial losses
Large Independent Group Practice	■ Overhead costs and financial risk spread among more physicians ■ Clinical synergies ■ Referral opportunities	■ Reduced independence ■ Reduced governance role ■ Liability for group financial and clinical performance
Employee Status	■ Low financial risk ■ Guaranteed paychecks ■ Relief from practice administration	■ Limited income growth potential ■ Little independence or control ■ Future tied to organization's success

Group Practice Questionnaire

Use the following questionnaire to gather information about each practice you consider. By accumulating the same information on each, you can compare using the same criteria.

General Information:

Date: _____

Name of Group: _____

Office Address: _____

Telephone: _____

Addresses of Satellite Offices:_____

Name of person to contact for future information:_____

Home Number: _____

Group Structure:

What is the legal structure of the group?

❏ Partnership

❏ Professional Corporation

❏ Limited Liability Corporation

❏ Individuals sharing space

Single or Multi specialty?_____

Who are the group's partners and/or principal stockholders?

Name: _____ Age: ____ Gender:____ Specialty: _____

Name: _____ Age: ____ Gender:____ Specialty: _____

Name: _____ Age: ____ Gender:____ Specialty: _____

Who are the employed physicians?

Name: _____ Age: ____ Gender:____ Specialty: _____

Name: _____ Age: ____ Gender:____ Specialty: _____

Name: _____ Age: ____ Gender:____ Specialty: _____

Are there physicians planning to retire? If so, what is the expected date(s) of retirement?

_____

Are there plans to increase the size of the group?

_____

What is the ultimate goal regarding size?

_____

What makes up the group's geographic market area? (Define by counties, miles, etc.)

_____

What is the population of the group's market area?

_____

How many physicians in my specialty, not associated with this group, practice in this market area?

_____

Area Hospitals:

List hospitals where group members have staff privileges.

Name:_____ # of beds:_____

Name:_____ # of beds:_____

Are there other hospitals in the area?_____

Does the group place restriction on having privileges at other hospitals?_____

Buy-In Opportunities

Does the group offer partnership to all physician employees? _____

What are the criteria for partnership? _____

    Number of years of employment required_____

    Is buy-in required? _____

    Are the buy-in requirements written into the original employment contract?_____

Practice Styles

What is the ethical orientation of the group (i.e., abortions, birth control, euthanasia, etc.)?

_____

Is there a feeling of compatibility and cooperation among group physicians?_____

Are all group members Board Certified? _____

Do any group members have a particular skill or certification that sets them apart from other specialists in the same field? If so, what are these skills?

_____

Are academic appointments encouraged? _____

Are there constraints placed on time spent in teaching activities? _____

Do any group members have academic appointments? _____

Are members involved in medical society activities? _____

Do any of the physicians have personal or practice problems or limitations of which you should be aware?

_____

How many physicians have left the group in the last three years?

_____

Were they employees or partner physicians?

_____

What were their reasons for leaving? _____

Will you have the opportunity to meet with the other physicians in the group before making a decision?

_____

Social Interactions

Do the physicians seem to have a good relationship with each other? _____

Is socializing expected or discouraged among physicians? _____

Do spouses socialize with each other? _____

Have you and your spouse met the spouses of the group's physicians? _____

How does your spouse feel about the physicians spouses he/she has met? _____

_____

Do any of the physicians have personal/social problems of which you are aware? _____

_____

Income Distribution

How is practice income distributed?

    ❑ *Equally*

    ❑ *Based on productivity*

❏ *Based on formula. If formula, what factors are used to determine income?*

_____

What method is used to allocate expenses?
   ❏ *Income and expenses shared equally*
   ❏ *Income and expenses based on productivity*
   ❏ *Income based on productivity, expenses shared equally*
      (Read Income Distribution, above, to interpret the answers to these questions.)

Office Facilities

*What was your first impression of the office appearance?*_____

_____

*How long has the group practiced at this address?*_____

*How many square feet are there in the facility?*_____

What ancillary services are provided in office? _____ ❏ *X-ray?* ❏ *Laboratory?*

How accessible is the practice location to patients? _____

*Are parking facilities adequate? If not, what plans exist to improve this?*_____

Will you have your own consulting office? _____

*How many exam rooms will you have?*_____

If there are satellite locations, are the physicians rotated through each location? _____

*What is the rotation schedule?*_____

Is the office clean? _____ *Well organized?*_____ *Well equipped?*_____

Are there plans for future expansion? _____

Is the size of the reception area adequate? _____

Is there adequate seating in the exam rooms? (Three seats per exam room is average.) _____

If your specialty requires special equipment, is it available? _____

Is the facility owned by the group, by the physicians personally, or leased from another entity?

_____

What is the distance to hospital(s)? _____

Is the practice in a high growth area or in a declining neighborhood? _____

What days and hours are the offices open? _____

Group Governance

How are decisions made within the group?
- ❏ *Majority vote?*
- ❏ *Governing board?*
- ❏ *Senior physicians?*
- ❏ *Informal clique?*

Who makes day-to-day decisions vs. long-term decisions or changes? _____

Is there an office manager/administrator? _____

To whom does this person report? _____

Are there regular business meetings? _____

How often are they held? _____

Are all physicians required to attend? _____

Office Personnel

How many employees in the practice? _____ *Clinical* _____ *Administrative* _____

What is the staff-to-physician ratio? _____

Are physician extenders used? _____ *How many P.A.s* _____ *Nurse Practitioners* _____

Does each physician have a personal clinical assistant? _____

Does the office appear over-or under-staffed? _____

How are patients treated by the staff? _____

Does the staff seem efficient, courteous and professional? _____

How many staff members have left voluntarily within the last year? _____

What were the reasons they left? (Ask staff members.) _____

_____

_____

How many staff members have been terminated? _____

Have they been replaced? _____

Is there good communication between staff and physicians? _____

Financial Overview:

Total charges last year: _____

Adjusted charges last year (after contractual write-offs, e.g., Medicare and managed care, etc.):

_____

Total collections, same period: _____

Total expenses: _____

Percent of total expenses for personnel wages: _____

Percent of total expenses for rent/mortgage expense: _____

Total accounts receivable: _____

Total dollars of A/R over 90 days: _____ *Percent of total A/R:* _____

Does the practice have an operational budget? _____

How does it compare with actual figures? _____

Does the group review financials together every month? _____

What reports will be provided to you? _____

What is the fee schedule? _____

Do all physicians use the same fee schedule? _____

Is billing and collections done in-house? _____

If not, how is it handled? _____

Is the practice computerized? _____

What software is used for practice management? _____

Who handles the payables? (office manager, accountant, other) _____

Who signs the checks? _____

Managed Care/Medicare Participation

Are all physicians participating in Medicare? _____

What percentage of practice is Medicare? _____ Medicaid?_____

How many managed care contracts does the group have?_____

What percentage of total patients are on managed care plans?_____

How many plans have at least 20 percent of the group's patient base? _____

Does any MCO have more than 20 percent of the group's patient base?_____

    Which ones? _____

Does the group have any capitated contracts?_____

How is information about each managed care contract tracked? _____

Does becoming a part of this group make you eligible to see patients on these contracts immediately?

_____

Patient Distribution

How are new patients distributed if no preference is given? _____

How is the patient load distributed?_____

How are managed care patients distributed in a group contract?_____

In a single specialty group, how are the unusual cases distributed?_____

Who sees nursing home patients?_____

What is the current call schedule rotation?_____

Malpractice Issues

What has been the group's malpractice experience? _____

Are any malpractice suits pending?_____

Are any considered having merit? _____

Are any liabilities retroactive?_____

CHAPTER 4

Tax and Licensing Requirements

Applying for State License and Provider Numbers

Once you have selected the location of your practice, you should begin the process of applying for the proper state licenses and provider numbers. You must also apply for certain federal and state tax identification numbers. Listed below are the most commonly required licenses and tax numbers. Check with the state government where you will practice to find out if there are other state-specific requirements.

State Medical License

Call the State Board of Medical Examiners to obtain the necessary forms and a list of any backup documents you will need to apply for your state license.

Medical Staff Privileges

Before you are cleared for medical staff privileges, you must have your state license. Visit each hospital in the area where you need to obtain staff privileges. Complete the necessary credentialing forms and collect any other documents you may need for admitting privileges. If you are joining a group practice and need to be on call, you can sometimes get temporary privileges until you have received your license.

Federal Narcotics License/Drug Enforcement Agency Number

If you currently have a DEA number, you must notify the DEA authorities of your new address. If you have never had a DEA number, you will need to write to the Department of Justice at the following address to obtain a license to dispense narcotics:

U.S. Department of Justice
Drug Enforcement Agency
Central Station
P.O. Box 28083
Washington, D.C. 20038-8083
202 307 7255

State Narcotics License

Some states will also require you to have a state narcotics license. Check to see if the state where you will be practicing requires a state DEA license in addition to the federal license.

Universal Provider Identification Number (UPIN)

The Health Care Financing Administration (HCFA) assigns every physician a Universal Provider Identification Number (UPIN). They will assign you this number when you apply for a Medicare Provider number. No extra forms are required for this.

In the latter part of 1996, HCFA is planning to discontinue the use of UPINs and begin instead a National Provider Identifier (NPI) program. They will assign you an NPI number that will replace your UPIN number if one has already been assigned. If you have not received a UPIN number by late 1996, they will most likely assign you the new NPI number instead.

Write to the Health Care Financing Administration and request any information available for a new physician.

Health Care Financing Administration
P.O. Box 26676
Baltimore, MD 21207
410 786 3000

HCFA has regional offices in every state. These can be found in the telephone directory in the blue pages titled "Government Listings."

Medicare Provider Number

If you are starting your own practice and you will be providing medical services to Medicare recipients, you will need to apply for a provider number. The Medicare program has two parts. Part A covers hospital services, and Part B covers physician services. If you already have a Medicare provider number and you are moving to another state, you will be assigned a new provider number for that state.

Each year, HCFA contracts with an insurer in each state to be the payer and administrator of Medicare claims in that state. You can learn who the Part B Medicare carrier is in your state by asking a local physician or office manager. (Do not get this information from the hospital. Hospitals often have a different carrier for Part A claims.) You will need to contact that carrier to obtain your Medicare provider number. If you are unable to find out who the Part B carrier is in your area, call HCFA at the number provided above.

You will need your state medical license to obtain your Medicare provider number.

Medicaid Provider Number

If you will be treating recipients of Medicaid services, you will also need a Medicaid provider number. You will obtain your Medicaid number from HCFA when you apply for a Medicare number.

If you are joining a group practice or becoming an employee of a hospital, your Medicare and Medicaid provider numbers will be linked with a group number for that group or employer. Your employer will help you in obtain your provider number.

You will keep the same Medicare and Medicaid numbers as long as you practice in the same state. If you change your address to another location within the state, you need only notify the carrier of your new address. If you move out of state, you will need a new number. Notification of address changes should be made well in advance to assure that your reimbursement is not delayed.

Retired Railroad Employees' Coverage

Travelers Insurance Company covers all retired railroad employees no matter where these retirees live. Once Travelers assigns a provider number, it stays the same regardless of where you practice.

Business License

Before you open your own office, you will need a business license. This will be either a city license or a county license, depending on where your practice is located. If you are within the city limits, go to the city hall to purchase your license. If your office is outside the city limits, you will most likely need to apply at the county courthouse for your license. In rare instances, you will need both a city and a county license. The cost of a license varies by city and by state, but will likely be between $100 and $300. A business license must be renewed every year.

Laboratory License

In October 1988, the federal government passed the Clinical Laboratories Improvement Act (CLIA). This act became effective in September of 1992 and requires that all physicians' office laboratories be licensed according to the complexity of the tests they perform. If you plan to do *any* laboratory testing on site, you will need a CLIA number.

Following is a list of the different levels of office laboratories and the tests that each category includes. Determine what tests you will be performing in your office, and apply for the appropriate level of license. Costs are involved in having an in-office laboratory. Each level has a registration fee and an annual inspection fee. Other costs are in proportion to the level of the laboratory and the annual test volume.

CLIA '88 Test Categories

Waived

Dipstick/Tablet Urinalysis
Ovulation Test Kits
Urine Pregnancy Tests
Sed Rates (manual)
Fecal Occult Blood
Glucose Meters
Manual Hematocrit
Hemoglobin (CuSO4)
Streptococcus Group
Helicobacter Pylori
Total Cholesterol
HDL Cholesterol
Triglycerides
Glucose

PPM (Physician-Performed Microscopy)

Wet Mounts
KOH Preps
Pinworm Preps
Fern Tests
Post-Coital Qualitative Exam
Urine Sediment Exam

Moderately Complex

Most Hematology Instruments
Manual Diff/Limited ID
Most Chemistry Tests
Urine Culture/Colony Count Only
Gram Stain/Urethral, Cervical for GC
Throat Screen/Hemo, Bacitracin, SSA
GC Screen/Gram Stain, Oxidase
Rapid Kits/Mono, Strep, Chlamydia

Highly Complex

Manual Cell Counts
Manual Diff/Complete ID
Some Esoteric Chemistry Tests
Urine Culture/Organism Identification
Gram Stain/Any Other Source
Throat Culture
GC Culture/Organism Identification
Antibiotic Susceptibility Testing

CLIA '88 Fees

Laboratory Schedule	Annual Test Volume	Number of Specialties	Registration Fee ($)	Accreditation Fee ($)	HCFA Inspection Fee ($)	Accreditation Validation Fee ($)
A Low Volume	<2000	Not specified	100	100	300	Not specified
A	2-10,000	3 or less	100	100	840	42
B	<10,000	4 or more	100	100	1120	56
C	10-25,000	3 or less	100	100	1400	70
D	10-25,000	4 or more	350	100	1645	82
E	25-50,000	Not specified	350	350	1890	95
F	50-75,000	Not specified	350	350	2135	107
G	75-100,000	Not specified	350	350	2380	119
H	100-500,000	Not specified	600	600	2625	131
I	500-1,000,000	Not specified	600	600	2870	141
J	1,000,000 or more	Not specified	600	600	Calculation required	Calculation required

Tax Identification Numbers

Employer Identification Number (EIN)

As an employer, you will need an Employer Identification Number (EIN). All correspondence with the IRS and all tax payments must reference this EIN. To apply for an EIN, you will need Form SS-4 which may be obtained at any IRS or Social Security Administration office. You will find the telephone number and address for the IRS Service Center nearest you in the telephone book under the State and/or Federal Government listings (blue pages). Once the application form has been completed and mailed, it takes approximately five weeks to receive your EIN. You may also apply for the EIN number by phone and receive the number immediately. Complete the Form SS-4 before you call the IRS Service Center for your state. When you obtain a number over the phone, you must mail in or FAX the completed Form SS-4 within 24 hours.

When you apply for an EIN number, the IRS will send you a book of payment coupons (Form 8109) that you will use when depositing your withholding taxes.

State Tax Identification Number

You may also need to apply for a State Tax Number. Check with your accountant to be certain you have all the required identifying numbers.

Resources

- Health Care Financing Administration
  P.O. Box 26676
  Baltimore, MD 21207

- U.S. Department of Justice
  Drug Enforcement Agency
  Central Station
  P. O. Box 28083
  Washington, D.C. 20038-8083
  202 307 7255

CHAPTER 5

Society Memberships/Practice Affiliations

Medical Society Membership

Membership in various medical societies, although not required for the practice of medicine, may be of benefit to the physician for information and networking. Annual fees range from $100 to more than $1,000 for membership in these associations. In the practice start-up phase, you will need to conserve cash; therefore, you will want to decide which of these affiliations will be most beneficial for you and your practice. Payment of these dues is often a benefit of group practice or employment.

The following associations are worth your consideration:

- *The American Medical Association* provides the physician a source of help and information about every aspect of the practice of medicine no matter where his practice is located. You do not have to be a member of the AMA to receive information or attend AMA-sponsored seminars. However, you will receive a discount on seminars, publications, and other services offered through the AMA if you are a member.

- *Local medical societies* (city and/or county) provide insights into the local politics of medicine and allow the physician to share ideas and information with other physicians practicing in the area.

- Your *national and/or state specialty association* will provide educational opportunities and information about your particular specialty and allow you to interact with physicians who share the same specialty-specific concerns.

- Becoming involved in *local civic groups* such as the Rotary Club, Kiwanis, Civitans, etc., provides many marketing opportunities. These groups allow the physician opportunities for meeting potential patients, and business persons who will be helpful in promoting the practice. Offering to speak to or for such groups present excellent marketing opportunities.

Other Practice Affiliations

Managed Care Organizations

When you have an address for your practice, begin completing applications for participation in various managed care plans. This process is often lengthy. It will be beneficial if you can begin to see managed care patients as soon as you open your office.

Before you attempt to participate in every plan available, do some investigative work. If you are a specialist, ask the primary care physicians in the area what plans they belong to and which ones have the best reputation and the most patients. To receive referrals, participating in the same plans as the primary care providers is necessary.

If you are joining a group practice, discuss managed care participation with the Medical Director or Office Manager. The applications will most likely be completed for you. However, you will need to provide all the necessary information to complete the forms. This information includes, but is not limited to, medical license, Board Certification, DEA number, hospital participation, and malpractice insurance.

Be sure you read the section on managed care in Chapter 13 before you enter the managed care arena.

Call Group Affiliation

A major hurdle in solo practice is finding other physicians in your specialty with whom to share call. You will need to talk with other physicians to see if there is an opportunity to join an existing call group. It may be necessary for you to take the initiative and start a new group. As a solo physician, look for every opportunity to share call with other physicians. Otherwise, you will have little opportunity for leisure or family time.

Physician Referral Service

Many hospitals have a physician referral service. Contact the hospital(s) where you will be practicing to see if such a service exists. Request that you be added to the referral list for your specialty. These referral services often limit the number of physicians in each specialty. So start right away to sign up, or be put on a waiting list if necessary. Ask whether they handle the referrals on a rotating basis or whether they give each patient a list of available physicians.

Emergency Room Coverage

Although the hospital in your area may have full-time emergency room coverage, there may be opportunities for you to work extra hours. If you are interested in "moonlighting," contact the ER Director at each hospital to see if such opportunities exist. If you are joining a group practice, check your contract to be sure there are no restrictions concerning employment outside the group.

CHAPTER 6

Office Accounting Procedures

Choosing a Computer System

Medical practices today are facing an environment of ever-increasing complexity in patient management and third party payment administration. To offset those complexities and reduce overhead costs, more practices are choosing to automate and integrate billing, accounting, medical record keeping, and appointment scheduling. Computerized practices are generally more efficient and have better internal controls.

The arrival of managed care has made using computers in the medical practice not only helpful, but essential. The volume of reports and other statistical data requested by managed care organizations can only be handled by a computerized practice management system.

Selecting a computer system for a medical practice requires time and effort on the part of the buyer. If you are unfamiliar with computers, you may choose to contract with a computer consultant before making this important investment. Consider using an independent consultant who is not associated with a firm that sells computer hardware or software.

If you elect to conduct your own research on a practice management system, remember that a management system is only as good as the information it gives you. At the end of this chapter we have provided a checklist of basic functions and reports that you should obtain from any practice management software you select. The second part of the checklist pertains to the tracking and administration of managed care plans, another essential function. These managed care tracking functions are not usually provided as a part of basic office management software but can be purchased as an added module. Before you make your final software selection, ask specific questions about the types and cost of managed care software that will interface with your system.

Training and ongoing support are important in vendor selection. Your new employees may not be familiar with the software you choose. Be sure that the training period is adequate and that provisions are made for staff turnover.

Most medical software systems are suitable for general, family and specialty practices. A good basic system ranges in price from $1,500 to $10,000. Compare the features and benefits of several packages. Then, decide for yourself which is most cost-effective based on your particular need. A checklist of computer functions to look for can be found in Chapter 10.

Establishing a Fee Schedule

There are various methods for establishing and reviewing fees in a medical office.

- Obtain fee information from other practices in your specialty, in your area. It is important that your fees be comparable.

- Refer to publications such as *The Physician's Fee Guide or Annual Physicians Fee Reference Book* available in most medical book stores.

- Use the Resource-Based Relative Value Scale (RBRVS) compiled by the federal Health Care Financing Administration (HCFA).

The Medicare fee schedule has been based on the RBRVS system since 1992. Most indemnity insurers and managed care organizations are beginning to base their reimbursement on this system as well.

RBRVS in a Nutshell

In the development of the RBRVS system, HCFA took more than 7,000 Current Procedural Terminology (CPT) codes to which they assigned a Relative Value Unit (RVU).

Each RVU has three components:

- Work RVU

- Overhead RVU

- Malpractice RVU

Added together, these equal the total RVU.

Recognizing that the cost of practicing medicine varies in different parts of the country, HCFA assigned a Geographic Practice Cost Index (GPCI) to each component of the RVU for each CPT code.

The total RVUs are multiplied by a standard conversion factor. Medicare has established a conversion factor for surgery, another for primary care services, and a third for non-surgical services. The 1996 conversion factors are as follows:

- Surgery $40.7986

- Non-Surgical $34.6293

- Primary Care $35.4173

NOTE: The Relative Value Units are reviewed and increased from time to time. Medicare may increase or lower the conversion factors each year based on the Medicare Volume Performance Standard (MVPS). The formula for establishing a new MVPS is very convoluted and not critical to understand. For the complete formula, refer to the Federal Register dated December 31, 1991, available in your local library.

The Complete RBRVS Formula

(Work RVU X Work GPCI) + (Overhead RVU X Overhead GPCI) + (Malpractice RVU X Malpractice GPCI) X the conversion factor = Total Fee

Example: CPT code 39502, Repair of a Hiatal Hernia, in Brownsville, Texas

Code 39502, Repair of Hiatal Hernia   Locality: Brownsville, TX

$$\frac{13.80}{\text{Work RVU}} \qquad \frac{1,008}{\text{Work GPCI}} \qquad = 13.841$$

$$\frac{12.57}{\text{Overhead RVU}} \qquad \frac{1,094}{\text{Overhead GPCI}} \qquad = 13.751$$

$$\frac{2.58}{\text{Malpractice RVU}} \qquad \frac{1,025}{\text{Malpractice GPCI}} \qquad = 2.644$$

Establishing your fees on the RBRVS system is the method of choice. Since HCFA has already established the RVUs for each CPT code, using the Medicare fee schedule to establish your fees is very simple. However, you will want to increase the conversion factor or simply increase the Medicare fee schedule by 25 percent to 30 percent, depending on what other physicians in your area are charging for the same services.

For example, if your competitor charges $1,600 for CPT code 39502 (Repair of a Hiatal Hernia) and the 1996 Medicare Fee for Code 39502 in your area is $1,233.59, you can increase the Medicare fee by 25 percent (approximately $300), set your standard fee at $1,550, and still be competitive in your area.

Cost of Providing a Service Versus Practice Fees

No matter how you set your fees, you cannot afford to deliver a service for a fee that is less than your cost of providing the service.

It is a fact that HCFA took the cost of providing a service into account when they established the overhead RVU for each service. However, HCFA's opinion of a reasonable profit margin and a physician's view of a reasonable profit margin are different. You must be aware of what your supplies cost to assure that your fees will provide you with a reasonable profit/salary after the bills are paid.

Purchasing Supplies

The first step in developing an organized purchasing system is to centralize the ordering process. Assign *one* person to be responsible for ordering supplies. In a new office, your Office Manager/ Office Assistant should order supplies. Having one person in charges eliminates duplicate orders, adds objectivity, and prevents having sales representatives talk to more than one person. The employee in charge of purchasing becomes familiar with supplies and prices and thus shops around for the best prices. Centralized ordering will also allow the purchaser to establish the quantity of each supply used over a given time, e.g., monthly, etc. These usage guidelines allow development of an inventory process that will reduce unnecessary inventory and control "panic orders" that increase expenses.

Use a simple steno pad as an order book. Each employee who needs supplies or uses the last of the current inventory will list the item in the order book. The Office Manager will order supplies based on what is written in the book. Use of an order log or order sheets may also be established.

Purchasing Tips:

- Create vendor files by company name and file all invoices and statements in chronological order. File the folders in alphabetical order.

- Be familiar with price breaks for regularly used items so that you can order in quantities that provide the best price.

- Purchase office supplies at local office supply discount stores instead of ordering by telephone from an office supply business. You can save up to 50 percent on some items this way.

- Every six months, check the prices you pay for standard items and compare vendor prices. Ask for competitive bids from three different vendors.

- Ask for a 45-day payment window.

- Negotiate!

Accounts Payable

If your office manager or assistant already has experience with accounting software, you may choose to purchase an accounting package that will produce a general ledger, income and expense statements and write checks. However, unless you have experienced personnel, adding this component later is best. The following information pertains to the establishment of a manual accounting system.

Chart of Accounts

Your accountant will help you establish a chart of accounts. Make sure the list is not too cumbersome. The chart of accounts is simply a list of numbers that identify each category of expense in your practice. This information is necessary for the accountant to allocate your expenses properly for tax purposes and cost accounting.

As an example, assume that the account number for medical supplies is 105. A check is written to XYZ Supply Company for hypodermic needles. The check should be made out to XYZ Company in the proper amount, and the account Number 105 should be written in red ink on the check stub. This number tells the accountant that the check to XYZ was for ***medical supplies***. For your internal use, the invoice numbers you are paying should also be listed on the stub.

It should be the responsibility of the person writing the checks to determine the account number to put on the check stub. The accountant cannot do this accurately because he or she may not know what supplies XYZ Company sells. Correct allocation of expenses is important. Keep a copy of the chart of accounts available for ready reference.

Paying Bills

The accounts payment process works best if bills are paid only once each month. Never pay bills in less than 30 days from the date of purchase unless you get a substantial discount for early payment. Keep the money in your bank working for you as long as possible, not in the vendor's bank earning interest.

Pay bills from invoices, not from vendor statements. Vendors seldom have the same billing cycle you have. If you make payment from a statement, you may mistakenly pay an invoice twice.

The Payment Process

At the same time each month, follow this routine for paying bills:

- Collect all the invoices you have received from a vendor in the previous 30 days. Check to make sure that the person receiving the goods has initialed the invoice to show that all goods ordered were received and in the proper quantities. Total the invoices and write a check for this amount.

- Write every invoice number you are paying and the amount on the check stub. Do not forget to put the chart of account number on the check and the check stub.

- Staple the invoices together, mark them "paid," and write the date and check number on them. You may want to buy a rubber stamp for this purpose.

- File the paid invoices in the vendor folder for that company. Keep only the invoices for the current year in your folder. At the end of each year, the invoices should be filed with other accounting papers for that year.

Establishing a workable accounts payable system at the start of your practice is critical. Accurate tracking of supply costs reduces overspending and panic buying, provides information needed for budgeting and forecasting, and gives the accountant the information necessary to prepare financial statements and tax returns.

CHAPTER 7

Choosing Your Advisors

Why Have Advisors?

In entering the practice of medicine, you will need local advisors to help you with various legal and accounting procedures. Rather than solicit advice from friends, family or others, you will be better served if you select an attorney and an accountant in the very beginning. You may want to seek recommendations from other physicians concerning these advisors.

An attorney will help you set up the legal structure of your practice and provide advice on a special-purpose basis. Use only attorneys who understand and have experience in health care law. There are more laws, statutes and legislation governing the practice of medicine now than ever before. Experienced, competent, and above all current advice is very important.

Using a capable accountant to assist in setting up your practice will assure that the practice provides you with the best tax advantages and flexibility. The accountant should also assist you in setting up your accounting system, establishing internal controls and preparing an operating budget.

Interview each attorney and accountant. Once you are convinced that the candidates have the experience you need, determine whether you can establish a rapport with them individually, and if they can work with each other. If communications are not good, there will be disagreements and misunderstandings. Choose these advisors with great care and forethought. An accountant you are happy with may recommend an attorney, or vice versa.

How to Select an Advisor

Following are suggestions for securing a professional advisor:

- Personal interview
- Check with the following references
  - Colleagues
  - Friends and associates
  - Local medical society
  - Local CPA society
  - Local bar association
  - Associations for professional business consultants

Selecting an Advisor

Use the following checklist when interviewing potential advisors.

- Qualifications of advisor matches your practice needs.

- Advisor has experience working for doctors, especially in your specialty.

- The advisor is certified or licensed.

- The advisor has provided references whom you have researched and received positive recommendations.

- The fee or method of payment is satisfactory and is to be one of the following:
  - Monthly retainer
  - Per hour
  - Commission

- The advisor's philosophy correlates with yours (e.g., conservative versus risk-taking, etc.)

- He is sensitive to your level of business expertise.

- Your personal and professional goals and objectives interface well with the advisor's.

- Vested or conflicting interests of the advisor have been identified.

- The advisor's availability is sufficient for your needs.

- The advisor can meet the timetable you have established.

- He is willing to sign a contract, if required.

- The advisor is conveniently located.

- The advisor will follow up on any recommendations to assure that they are carried out; such follow up will be part of the cost.

When to Use an Advisor

An advisor can be helpful to assist you in the following areas:

- Practice management functions
  - Income tax planning and preparation
  - Audits
  - Systems revisions or enhancements
  - Problems with office personnel, collections, expenses
  - Reviewing managed care contracts
  - Establishing a fee schedule

- Formation of a group practice, partnership, or corporation
  - Legal advice
  - Accounting advice

Advisors to be Considered

The following professionals may provide vital assistance to you in their areas of specialization:

- Accountant
- Lawyer

- Banker

- Investment counselor

- Management consultant

- Insurance broker or salesperson

- Real estate broker

While attorneys and practice management consultants will assist you with occasional situations in your office, your accountant will have a continuous relationship with the practice. Perhaps one of the most important characteristics to look for should be how well he relates to you. This relationship requires a high level of trust and understanding.

Selecting an Accountant

The person you hire to give you accounting advice does not necessarily have to be a Certified Public Accountant (CPA). However, selecting the right accountant should be based on the same criteria as selecting a physician, technical knowledge and a personal relationship. Select an accountant on a trial basis. The following descriptions will help you in differentiating various accounting professionals and the roles they fill:

Certified Public Accountant. A CPA will have the highest level of expertise in the field of accounting. Choose someone with experience in dealing with medical practices, corporations, and tax planning. CPAs generally charge by the hour. Some CPAs are a part of accounting firms; others have solo practices.

Bookkeeping/Accounting Services. Bookkeeping services are available in almost every location. Typically, they can prepare monthly financial statements based on cash receipts and disbursements that you provide. Bookkeepers can probably prepare income tax returns, but they may be limited in how much tax planning and/or business advice they can provide. Bookkeeping services generally do not have to meet professional or state licensing requirements and are less expensive than accounting firms or CPAs.

Practice Office Management Services. These companies not only do accounting and tax work for the practice but may also perform such services as hiring employees, maintaining bank accounts, writing checks, billing and collecting accounts receivable, purchasing office and medical supplies, and contracting for laboratory or janitorial services. Practice management firms can be very helpful in the start-up phase of your practice to assist you in setting up your overall business operations. Carefully check the qualifications and reputation of the company you are considering. The fees associated with this type of service are often high.

Regardless of whether you choose an accountant, bookkeeper, or practice consultant, be sure they will provide the following services:

- Assist you, your spouse and medical assistant to understand and establish a basic budget.

- Determine the need for periodic reviews of practice and set these up.

- Train your office assistant to do simple bookkeeping or accounting tasks.

- Conduct regular audits of the accounts receivable and accounts payable.

- Reconcile the bank statement.

- Explain the IRS laws and penalties.
- Instruct you on how to keep adequate records on contributions, real estate, sales tax, interest and dividends received, etc.
- Prepare monthly or quarterly financial statements.
- Prepare payroll and payroll taxes.
- Meet with you or your assistant regularly to compare budget with actual expenditures and make recommendations for improvement.

Other advisors will include your banker and your insurance agent. By this time you may already have established a line of credit or a business loan through a local bank. We suggest that you go through the same bank for all your banking needs. Consolidating your needs with one bank or banker will help you to establish a relationship of mutual trust and benefit. A bank that is locally owned and operated may also be of benefit to you. Local banks are generally more receptive to making unsecured loans to local businesspeople.

Selecting an Insurance Agent/Broker

Choosing an insurance agent or broker can be more critical than you might think, as you will devote a considerable part of your operating budget to health, liability and Workers' Compensation insurance premiums. Seek recommendations for this advisor from your accountant, attorney, or from other physicians in the area.

Selecting a Practice Management Consultant

Many physicians and physician groups go through the entire practice cycle without ever seeking the assistance of a "Practice Management Consultant." Unfortunately, these physicians probably spend many hours of their own valuable time and efforts on projects that a consultant could handle in a fraction of the time.

A physician new to practice, in particular, will benefit greatly by using an experienced consultant. Besides offering advice and organizing the practice set up, the experienced consultant can develop policies and procedures manuals, fee schedules and job descriptions for the new practice.

When selecting the practice consultant, ask candidates for the names of other physicians whom the consultant has helped. Talking with these references provides a feel for the consultant's knowledge and the success of the projects in which he has assisted a physician.

Use a written agreement (between the physician and the consultant) listing, as specifically as possible, what you expect to be achieved. Corresponding to this list, the practice management consultant should state exactly what he will provide. The agreement should also establish the schedule for accomplishment of the work.

Practice management consultants are numerous. Your city's telephone directory will list consultants in your area. Ask for references!

Listed below are a few national companies you may wish to contact.

AMA Financing and Practice Services Division
200 North La Salle Street, Suite 500
Chicago, IL 60601
312 419 5042

Medical Group Management Association
104 Inverness Terrace East
Englewood, CO 80112-5306
303 799 1111

The Coker Group
3150 Holcomb Bridge Road, Suite 200
Norcross, GA 30071
800 345 5829
Max Reiboldt, CFO
Lauretta Mink, Vice President of Practice Services

CHAPTER 8

Identifying Insurance Requirements

Among the most crucial decisions you will make concerns the insurance coverage you purchase. Some types of insurance are required by state law, others by your hospital or managed care plans, and still others by your office or equipment leases. Following is a brief explanation of these types of insurance coverage.

Every medical employer carries some form of insurance in addition to professional liability coverage. This might include property insurance, commercial general liability insurance (CGL), life insurance, overhead disability insurance, Workers' Compensation insurance, group health insurance, and fidelity bond insurance that protects the practice if there is embezzlement.

Professional Liability Insurance

There are many different sources for purchasing malpractice insurance, including traditional insurance companies, physician-owned companies, self-insured companies, group purchasing programs, and risk retention groups. What is available to you depends largely upon how much coverage you plan to purchase and the vendors who are in your area. Not all carriers operate in every state.

Depending on your specialty, professional liability insurance may be your single highest expense. Some things to look for in choosing the carrier include the following:

- The company's financial condition. Litigation takes three to five years. Seek coverage from a company that is apt to be around to defend you.

- Risk management/loss prevention assistance and advice.

- A comprehensive policy. Make sure you know what it does and does not cover. Review a copy of the policy, paying particular attention to the exclusions.

- Experienced claim professionals and a strong legal network.

Following are points to consider when purchasing your coverage:

- Purchase adequate limits. Many physicians purchase coverage based on the minimum requirements of the hospital(s) in which they practice, usually $1,000,000 per occurrence and $3,000,000 aggregate. However, you do not want a single occurrence to exhaust the coverage under your policy. The aggregate should be two to three times your occurrence limit.

- Understand the claims made coverage and the importance of continuous coverage.

- The added expense of higher limits of liability may be cost effective for you.

- Name your professional corporation on your policy. Most legal actions will name both you and your corporation.

- Consider insuring the corporation separately. You can increase your available coverage for a fraction of the cost of increasing your individual limits.

- Make sure that nurses, professional assistants, nurse practitioners or midwives in your employ are properly covered.

Note: Most group practices have a group policy for professional liability coverage. If you are joining a medical group, they will most likely cover you under the group's policy. Your premiums may be a part of your compensation package. If you already have malpractice coverage that you will cancel when you join the group, you will need to purchase "tail coverage." This will cover any potential litigation stemming from actions prior to becoming a member of the group or an employee. Be sure you check with your group/employer to find out who is responsible for payment of the "tail coverage." Leave nothing to chance!

Standard Office Insurance

One way to purchase the protection you need for your office is to buy an Office Package. The standard office package usually includes the following coverages.

Property Insurance

You have just spent a considerable amount of money to purchase the furniture and equipment necessary to start your practice. Evaluate the cost to replace the tangible assets owned by the practice to determine the proper amount of insurance to purchase. Purchase an adequate amount of property insurance to replace furniture and equipment in the event they are destroyed. In addition to your fixed assets, include office supplies, medical supplies, medical books and journals, artwork, files and file contents.

You may purchase many options through your property insurance. Depending on where you are located, you may want to consider earthquake or flood coverage. They usually exclude these from property policies. Always request "special" or "all risk" coverage. Consider higher deductibles to reduce costs. Try to use companies rated "A" or better by A. M. Best.

Computer Coverage

Your property insurance will cover your computer hardware; however, you may wish to purchase additional coverage that includes loss due to power surges or loss of data. Consult your software vendor to see how much software insurance you need for licensed software.

Business Income Insurance

This coverage is important and inexpensive. Business interruption insurance is actually disability insurance for your office. If your office becomes inaccessible due to a covered property loss (e.g., fire, hurricane, etc.), this coverage will reimburse you for lost revenues, continuous expenses, and lost profit. You will want to ensure that the coverage includes funds for a temporary office, expediting expenses, advertising the new location to your patients, and the expenditures to move back into your office once the damage has been repaired.

Employee Dishonesty Insurance

This coverage protects you if there is employee theft or embezzlement of funds.

Equipment Breakdown Coverage

This insurance covers the cost to repair or replace equipment that may be a means of generating significant revenue to your practice. Coverage also includes lost revenue for the period the equipment is unusable.

Commercial General Liability Coverage (CGL)

The CGL policy is a comprehensive form of coverage that provides protection from lawsuits brought against you by third parties. A third person is any individual other than the policyholder, the insurance company, or persons specifically exempted from coverage under the policy. The policy typically includes personal injury, product liability, advertising liability and contractual liability. Look for policy limits of $1,000,000 to $5,000,000. The cost for the higher limits is often minimal.

You will also want to consider non-owned and hired automobile liability. Non-owned coverage would cover an employee's vehicle used for the business of the practice such as going to the bank or post office. Hired autos, of course, would cover rented automobiles. *It is important to note that this is liability coverage and covers only damages to a third party. It does not cover the employee's car or the rented automobile.*

Workers' Compensation Insurance

Workers' Compensation Insurance is mandatory in most states if you have three or more employees. Each state regulates benefits and costs, so most policies have identical coverage. Make sure the policy you purchase is covered by your state's insurance insolvency fund.

Premiums are based on payroll estimates for a twelve-month policy term, subject to a final audit to adjust for changes. All wages should be included in the payroll estimates, including bonuses. Overtime, however, may be adjusted to its regular time equivalent.

Following are other tips to consider before you purchase your insurance policies:

- Higher deductibles usually mean lower premiums.

- Avoid over buying. Expensive "add-ons" are unnecessary if you have good coverage on your basic policy.

- Select appropriate policy limits and buy larger amounts of protection when doing so is economical. Increasing your limits under a liability policy is usually cheaper than adding coverage under a second policy.

- Pay smaller claims yourself. This must be done legally, so consult with your insurance company on this option.

- Give prompt attention to any third party claim.

Whatever the type of insurance coverage you purchase, there is no substitute for risk management. Work with your insurer or agent to help you develop a sound loss prevention program for all forms of practice liability. Conducting a regular loss prevention inservice education program will keep your employees aware of the importance of loss prevention and on-the-job safety.

CHAPTER 9

Financing the Medical Practice

Financing Options

Considering that the average physician completes his training as a resident with an excess of $50,000 in debt and no assets, it is not surprising that nearly every new physician starts a medical practice with someone else's money. Further, as a result of health care reform, even established physicians are having some financial woes. This has made banks more cautious about new physician loans.

The cost of starting a new practice is estimated to be somewhere between $100,000 and $150,000, so the new physician is seeking a sizeable unsecured loan. Banking professionals regard more favorably a physician who displays sufficient understanding of the business aspects of operating a medical practice.

Writing the Business Plan

A business plan should be developed before the physician attempts to attain financing from a bank. An effective business plan will break out the components necessary to run a business. It will include items like a market analysis, location of the building, plans for any renovations, equipment needed for the office, insurance costs, pricing strategy, and financial projections. Unless you have an unusual amount of business acumen and experience in preparing business plans, you will presumably need the assistance of an accountant to develop your business plan. The new physician who approaches a bank or other lender with a well thought out business plan enhances his chances of receiving the needed resources.

A business plan will also give you a clear picture of what is really required to start a business. It will consist of the following components:

- Executive Summary
- Description of the business
- Analysis of the market and competition
- Equipment and furniture needs
- Practice proforma/cash flow projections
- Copy of the office lease agreement
- Advertising/marketing strategies
- Personal profile information or CV

A loan from a bank may be in the form of a lump sum or a line of credit. Establishing a line of credit will allow you to draw funds, in necessary increments, against a maximum amount. In the initial months of practice start-up, you will need to draw more funds, but as you begin to see patients and generate revenue, your requirements will decline. A line of credit has an added benefit in that you only pay interest on the amount you have used.

Banks are not the only available sources for funding a medical practice. The federally funded Small Business Administration (SBA) may be able to help. The SBA does not actually lend you the money, but it guarantees the lender that the loan will be repaid. To obtain an SBA loan, seek a financial institution that belongs to the SBA. The SBA will often guarantee the lender as much as 90 percent of the loan amount. The paperwork for an SBA loan is often burdensome. It is the federal government, not the bank, who decides who gets a loan.

However, the SBA has recently developed a new program for loans less than $100,000. In this new program, the banker actually decides who gets a loan based on the individual's credit history, character, and the projected income stream of the business.

Determining the Loan Amount

Before you decide the amount of the loan or line of credit for which you will apply, you must have some idea of the cost of setting up the practice. To determine these costs, begin with Step One, compiling a series of lists, as follows:

- The first list will be the furniture and equipment you will need to set up the office.

- The second list will consist of the small pieces of reusable office equipment you will need. This list will include staplers, trash bins, pencil sharpeners, tape dispensers, and the like.

- Your third list will be all the disposable office and medical supplies you will need for the first three months of operation.

Using your lists, determine the cost for each item and calculate a total cost for all your purchases. For accounting and budgeting purposes, the accountant will separate these items into capital and non-capital expenses.

Following is an example of items needed for furnishing and equipping a medical practice for one physician with three exam rooms and one procedure room. Prices are approximate based on research dated 1995.

Equipment Budget Checklist/Furniture and Equipment List (Sample)

1 Physician, 3 Exam Rooms, 1 Procedure Room

Phase I	Qty	Item	Unit Cost	Total Cost
CAPITAL		**MEDICAL EQUIPMENT**		
	3	Exam Tables	$637.00	$1,911.00
	1	Procedure table	$6,000.00	$6,000.00
	1	Hand-held pulse oximeter	$1,000.00	$1,000.00
	1	Autoclave	$1,745.00	$1,745.00
	1	Microscope	$875.00	$875.00
	1	EKG Machine	$2,750.00	$2,750.00
	1	Executive desk	$581.79	$581.79
	1	Credenza	$574.07	$574.07
	1	10 cu. ft. refrigerator (no frost), includes icemaker, delivery and installation	$649.00	$649.00
	1	Fax machine	$1,200.00	$1,200.00
	1	High-volume copy machine w/cabinet	$2,520.00	$2,520.00
	2	6-tier lateral file cabinet	$641.50	$1,283.00
		TOTAL CAPITAL		***$21,088.86***
NON-CAPITAL		**MEDICAL EQUIPMENT**		
	4	ENT wall unit	$225.00	$900.00
	4	Ophthalmoscope	$122.00	$488.00
	4	Otoscope	$66.00	$264.00
	4	Wall unit sphygmomanometer	$75.16	$300.64
	4	Outpatient exam light	$62.00	$248.00
	4	Midmark spin stool	$145.50	$582.00
	1	Two section x-ray viewbox	$199.00	$199.00
	2	Tycos stethoscope	$37.14	$74.28
	1	Mayo stands	$86.00	$86.00
	1	Eye chart	$3.50	$3.50
	1	Adult scale	$165.00	$165.00
	1	Double-lock narcotics cabinet	$149.00	$149.00
	1	Hand-held cobalt blue light	$15.00	$15.00
	1	Pelvic light	$81.00	$81.00
	1	Digital thermometers	$270.00	$270.00
	1	Pulmonary function unit	$125.00	$125.00
	1	Biohazard trash hamper	$74.00	$74.00
	1	Wheelchair	$175.00	$175.00
	1	EKG stand/utility cart	$130.00	$130.00

Equipment Budget Checklist/Furniture and Equipment List (Sample)

Continued

Phase I	Qty	Item	Unit Cost	Total Cost
		OFFICE FURNITURE		
	4	Point side chairs w/o arms	$159.90	$635.60
	4	Secretarial chairs	$158.21	$632.84
	1	Executive chairs	$361.60	$361.60
	2	Bookcases	$183.40	$366.80
	12	Reception chairs	$225.00	$2,700.00
	2	End tables	$142.50	$285.00
	1	Parson's table	$169.57	$169.57
	1	Break table	$169.85	$169.85
	1	Manager's desk	$407.57	$407.57
	1	Step stool w/ handle	$38.00	$38.00
		FIXTURES/ACCESSORIES		
	1	Outdoor combo ashtray & waste receptacle	$78.00	$78.00
		APPLIANCES/EQUIPMENT		
	1	Under-counter refrigerator	$149.97	$149.97
	1	Microwave w/ turntable	$139.97	$139.97
	1	Under cabinet coffee maker	$44.97	$44.97
	1	10-key calculator	$53.00	$53.00
	1	Video player & monitor	$399.92	$399.92
	1	Typewriter	$250.00	$250.00
		MISCELLANEOUS		
	1	Lantern-style flashlight	$16.97	$16.97
	1	Tool box w/assortment of tools	$39.97	$39.97
	4	Extension cords/surge protect	$25.00	$100.00
		TOTAL NON-CAPITAL		*$11,453.02*

Office Supply Budget Checklist (Sample)

Quantity	Item	Cost
1 Case	HCFA 1500 Claim Forms	40.00
1 Case	Copier/Fax Paper	50.00
1,000	Printed Billing Statements	300.00
6 Doz.	Pens & Pencils	10.00
1 Doz.	Calculator Paper Rolls	4.00
500	Patient Chart Folders	1,000.00
Pkg. 24	Post It Notes	15.00
6 Rolls	Celephane Tape	10.00
2 Boxes	Staples	3.00
12 Bxs.	Paper Clips (6 lg. & 6 sm.)	8.00
1 Box	Manila Envelopes	5.00
1 Box	Adhesive Labels	26.00
1 Doz.	Memo Pads	10.00
1 Box	Typewriter Ribbons	20.00
1 Box	Typewriter Correcting Tapes	20.00
1 Doz.	White Out Correction Fluid	8.00
3	Staplers	15.00
3	Staple Removers	6.00
3	Tape Despensers	15.00
3	Clip Boards	7.50
1 Box	Manila File Folders	10.00
1 Box	File Folder Index Sheets	5.00
1 Box	Hanging Folders	15.00
3 Bxs.	Year Labels	10.00
1 Set	Alpha Tabs (for chart folders)	50.00
2	2 Hole Punch	20.00
1	3 Hole Punch	15.00
3	Paper Clip Holders	7.00
COLUMN TOTAL		**$1,724.20**

Quantity	Item	Cost
2	Scissors	20.00
2	Desk Calendars	30.00
9	Letter Trays	40.00
3	Door Pockets	15.00
1	Appointment Book	20.00
1	Coil Pen (for reception desk)	5.00
1	Electric Pencil Sharpener	15.00
1 Doz.	Light Bulbs	15.00
1	Petty Cash Box	15.00
1	Bulletin Board	8.00
1 Box	Thumb Tacks	2.00
1 Box	Rubber Bands (assorted)	2.00
2	Stamp Pads	3.00
1	Wall Clock	15.00
2	Letter Openers	10.00
1	Expandable Paper Sorter	10.00
1 Doz.	Lined Pads (8.5 x 11)	10.00
2	Index Card File	40.00
3	Pen & Pencil Holders	10.00
1 Box	Floppy Disks	15.00
1	Liquid Glue Stick	3.00
1	Money Box w/ Lock	25.00
1	Step Stool	45.00
1 Each	Mop/Broom	10.00
1	Message Holder	6.00
6 Each	Highlighters/Wide Markers	12.00
3	Rulers	3.00
3 Bxs.	Binder Clips (assorted sizes)	15.00
GRAND TOTAL		**$2,056.50**

Medical Supply Budget Checklist

Item	Qty.	Price	Cost
INSTRUMENTS			
Blades & Handles			
Cervical Biopsy Punch			
Cervical Tenaculum			
Circumcision Clamp			
Cutaneous Punch			
Ear Curettes			
Ear Piercer			
Ear Spoon & Hook			
Ear Syringe			
Eye, Needle & Spud			
Fingernail Drill			
Finger Ring Cutter			
FORCEPS			
Dressing			
Ear			
Hemostatic			
Mosquito			
Splinter			
Sponge Holding			
Tissue			
Towel			
Uterine			
Hemorrhoidal Ligator			
I.U.D. Extractor			
Laryngoscopes			
Nail Clipper			
Nasal Specula			
Needle Holders			
Pelvimeter			
Rectal Probe & Hooks			
Rectal Specula			
Rectal Suction Tube			
Retractors			
Scapels, Disposable			
SCISSORS			
Bandage Dissecting			
Iris			
Operating			
Stitch			
Tuning Forks			
Uterine Curette			
Uterine Sounds			
Urethral Sounds			

Item	Qty.	Price	Cost
STERILIZATION, DISINFECTANTS, & CLEANERS			
Autoclave Test Record			
Air Deodorizers			
Dialdehyde Solution			
Disinfectant/Deodorant Spray			
Foam Surface Cleaners			
Germicidal Solution			
Heat Sealer			
Instrument Lubricant			
Instrument Sterilization Containers			
Sterilization Monitors, Strips/Tape/Sheets			
Sterilization Pouches/ Tubes/Wraps			
Sterilizer Forceps			
Sterilizing Record System			
Ultrasonic Cleaners			
Ultrasonic Solutions			
SYRINGES & NEEDLES			
Allergist Packs			
Destruction Devices			
Hypodermic Needles			
Special Procedure Needles			
Syringe/Needle Combinations			
SYRINGES			
Allergy			
Control			
Insulin			
Irrigation			
Tuberculin			
Utility			
Trays, Special Procedure			

Medical Supply Budget Checklist (continued)

Item	Qty.	Price	Cost
LABORATORY SUPPLIES			
Labels, Precut			
Latex Tubing			
Markers			
Media, Plated			
MICROSCOPE			
Cover Glasses			
Slides			
Mixer, Orbital Motion			
pH Paper			
PIPETTES			
Blood Diluting, RBC/WBC			
Lambda, Disposable			
Sahli			
Transfer			
Pipette Shaker/Washer			
Plastic Labware			
Potassium Analyzer			
Prothrombinmeter/Supplies			
Reagent Strips, Dip & Read			
Refractometer			
Refrigerator			
Rh View Box			
Rotator			
Sedimentation Apparatus			
Serology Analyzer			
Serum Separation Tubes			
Specimen Collectors, Urine/Feces			
Stains & Reagents			
Stool, Lab			
Thyroid Function Tester			
Timers Ty Systems, Lab			
TUBES			
Capillary			
Centrifuge			
Hematocrit			
Sedimentation			
Serum Separation			
Urinalysis Reagent Strips/Tablets			
Urinometer			
Water Bath			

Item	Qty.	Price	Cost

Medical Supply Budget Checklist (continued)

Item	Qty.	Price	Cost
DRESSINGS			
Adhesive Closures			
Adhesive Pads, Sterile			
Adhesive Strips, Patches, Spots			
Adhesive Tapes			
Adhesive Tapes Remover, Pads/Spray			
Ammonia Inhalant Pads			
Benzoin Spray			
Burn Spray			
Butterfly Closures			
Combine Dressings			
Conforming Bandages			
Cotton or Rayon Balls			
Cotton Rolls			
Elastic Tape			
Eye Pads			
First Aid Kit			
Gauze Bandages			
Gauze Dressings			
Gauze Packing Strips			
Gauze Sponges			
Incontinent Cleanser			
Lubricating Jelly			
Merthiolate Spray			
Non Adherent Dressings			
Ointment Dressings			
Petrolatum Gauze			
Adherent Wrap			
Spray On Dressings			
Topical Anesthetic Spray			
Topical Skin Freeze Spray			
Towelettes			
Transparent Dressing			
Tubular Gauze			
Wound Closure Strips			

Item	Qty.	Price	Cost
SUNDRIES			
Alcohol Dispenser			
Atomizer			
Bags, Doctors, Nurses, EMT			
Batteries, General Use			
Cotton Tipped Applicators			
Diaphragms			
Dialators, Rectal/Vaginal			
Disinfectant/Deodorant Spray			
Dressing Jars, SS or Glass			
Ear Basin			
Finger Cots			
Flashlights			
Forceps Jar			
Gloves, Examination/ Surgical			
Hand Lotion			
Instrument Trays, SS w/ Cover			
I.U.D.'s			
Labels			
Lubricating Jelly			
Markers, Waterproof			
Nebulizers			
Organizers & Bins			
Room Deoderizers			
Sanitary Napkins/Belts			
Sigmoidoscope Applicators			
Signs & Signage			
Silver Nitrate Applicators			
Soap, Lotion/Bar			
Straws, Drinking			
Sundry Jars w/ Lids, Labeled			
Tape Measures			
Tapewriter			
Thermometer Holder/ Sheaths			
Thermometers, Oral & Rectal			
Tubing, Latex			
Tongue Depressors			
Wood Applicators			

Medical Supply Budget Checklist (continued)

Item	Qty.	Price	Cost
ORTHOPEDIC			
Ankle Supports			
Ankle Wrap			
Arm Slings			
CAST			
Boots			
Padding			
Walking Heels			
Cervical Collar			
Clavicle Strap			
Colles Splint			
Elastic Bandages			
Felt			
Fiberglass Casts			
Finger Splints, Assorted			
Head Halter			
Knee Immobilizers			
Lumbosacral Support			
PLASTER			
Apron			
Bandages			
Knife			
Shears			
Splints			
Rib Belts			
Shoulder Immobilizer			
Casting System			
Traction Kit			
Tubular Bandages/ Stockingnette			
Wrist Supports			
PAPER & PLASTIC PRODUCTS			
Capes, Examination			
Cup Dispenser			
Cups, Paper & Plastic			
Drape Sheets			
Face Masks			
Facial Tissues			
Gowns, Examination			
Labels, Medical			
Lab Coat, Disposable			
Medicine Cups			
Office Coat, Disposable			
Patient Bib			
Pillow Cases			
Sheets, Paper			
Table Paper & Holder			
Toilet Tissue			
Towels, Paper/Dispenser			
Wash Cloths			

Item	Qty.	Price	Cost
BIOLOGICALS, INJECTABLES			
Biologicals			
Chemicals			
Injectables			
Liquids			
Ointments & Creams			
Tablets & Capsules			
Miscellaneous			
LABORATORY SUPPLIES			
Automatic Pipettors			
Bacteria Identification System			
BLOOD COLLECTION			
Chair			
Lancets			
Needles & Holders			
Prep Applicators			
Syringe/Needle			
Tourniquet			
Vacuum Tubes			
Blood Glucose Monitor/Strips			
Blood Grouping/Typing Strips			
Blood Grouping Slides			
Cervical Scraper			
Coagulating Cups/Tips			
Cytological Fixative			
Detergent, Laboratory			
DIAGNOSTIC SCREENING TESTS			
Gonorrhoea			
Meningitis			
Mononucleosis			
Occult Blood			
Pregnancy			
Rheumatoid Factor			
Rubella			
Sickle Cell			
Streptococcus			
Syphilis			
Flame Photometer			
Glucose Tolerance Test			
Hematocrit Tube Reader			
Hematocrit Tube Sealer			
Hemolysis Applicators			
Inoculating Loop & Holder			
Inoculating Loop Sterilizer			

Step Two will be preparation of the cash flow forecast and budget. The cash flow forecast will show how much revenue you expect to generate per month, during the first year. This forecast will allow the lender to calculate how much you will need monthly to draw against your credit line to cover your office and personal expenses.

By the time you reach the budget planning stage on your time line, you should have already selected your accountant. Using his expertise in this process will benefit you. The accountant may already have a "canned" budget for a new medical practice. While it may serve as a good starting place, be cautious about relying on it entirely. An accurate operating budget must be based on your particular specialty and the geographic area.

A budget is simply a plan. Your initial operating budget is a plan for how your practice will operate during your first year of practice. In an existing business, the operating budget is based partly on historical financial data and partly on forecasts for the future. For a new medical practice, there is no historical data, so the budget will be based on industry standards and a good deal of guesswork.

After you have completed your cash flow forecast and your operating budget, compile the other supporting documents for the business plan. Write your executive summary, then have all the information neatly prepared for presentation. The more professional your business plan looks, the more successful you will be in obtaining the credit you need.

CHAPTER 10

Leasing Space and Purchasing Equipment

Selecting an Office Location

The careful selection of your office location is critically important. Choose a geographic area that is convenient for the patients you will be serving and in line with your specialty. For example, if your specialty is pediatrics, a location in the suburbs may be more appropriate than one in the downtown office district. Location, not cost, should be the determining factor in an office lease. Remember that a lease is a binding agreement; you may be locked in for several years.

How much you are able to negotiate on the lease rate varies with supply and demand. If ample office space is available, you can probably negotiate an excellent deal. On the other hand, if only limited office space is available, the landlord will be much less willing to negotiate.

Set priorities for the items that are important to you in the contract and seek advice from your attorney before you sign. Obtain everything about your leasing arrangements in writing. Make no agreements based simply "on a handshake," regardless of whom your landlord will be. A well-written lease protects both the lessor and the lessee.

Below is a list of some considerations in office leasing that are most important to physicians.

What to Look for in an Office Lease

Location and Description of Space. Be sure you understand how the space is being measured, then measure it yourself. Hallway space is sometimes included in the square footage. Do not pay for space you cannot use.

Check to see if your rental agreement includes parking spaces. Find out how many and where they are. If your patients have no place to park, the office space is useless. A good "rule of thumb" measure is one parking space for every chair in your reception area.

Term. We recommend you sign a first lease for no more than three years. This will allow you enough time to give the locale a fair chance. A viable practice should begin to show strong profits by the third year. While a ten-year lease may feature an attractively low rent, getting out of it may be hard if you decided to move to another location.

Option to Renew. As an alternative to a long term lease, you might want to sign a three-year lease with two, three-year options to renew. These options should include any future rental increases in writing.

Rental. Know to whom the rent is payable. A landlord who lives halfway across the country is not likely to be as responsive to your requests for repairs and improvements as one who lives in the same town.

Escalation Clause. Even a three-year lease may have rental increases every year. These increases are usually based on the landlord's taxes and cost of operations, such as maintenance and utilities. Rent in commercial space is quoted as cost-per-square foot annually.

Damage Deposit. Find out how much of a damage deposit is required and if your deposit will earn interest. Be sure all repairs are made before you move in or that an appropriate clause noting the needed repairs is included in the lease. Most leases have some wording concerning the condition of the space after the lease has expired. Some state that "all leasehold improvements become the property of the landlord" or "the premises must be returned to their original condition." In either case, the tenant loses. You will either give up items you have installed, like sinks, cabinets, wallpaper and even expensive draperies, or you will have to resurface and repaint the walls. This can be very expensive if you decide to move.

Escape Clause. Be sure that your office lease contains an escape clause releasing you from your obligations should you lose your license or hospital privileges or become disabled. An escape clause should also be included to protect your estate in the event of your death.

Items and Services Furnished. Maintenance, security, repairs, lawn mowing, and snow removal all come under this category. Make no assumptions about anything. Any services furnished and costs covered must be itemized in the lease. Check out the credentials of the building maintenance service; be sure they are bonded. If you plan to see patients at nontraditional hours, be sure you know the hours of operation for the air conditioning, elevators and security. Be clear about the kind of signage you will be allowed or provided.

Insurance. Learn what kind of coverage the landlord has for accidents that may occur in the foyer, parking lot, and so forth. Check with your insurance agent to see if you need a supplemental policy for any gaps that may exist.

Remodeling and Redecoration. Does the lease agreement tell you how often your office will be repainted or the carpet replaced? How often does the landlord repaint or redecorate the common areas? Who pays for these improvements?

Subleasing. If you choose to move before your lease expires, will you be allowed to sublet your space? Does the lease restrict the sublet clause to certain kinds of businesses? While you want the sublet clause to be reasonable, you also want to assure that another tenant does not sublease space to an undesirable tenant.

Unfit for Occupancy. This clause usually covers storm damage and other acts of nature. However, you will want to assure that the lease covers other disruptions such as loss of heat or air conditioning. You may not be able to see patients for several days, and you want to be sure you do not have to pay rent for those days the space is uninhabitable.

Right of First Refusal. This clause states, "You will be offered the first opportunity to lease any additional space that becomes available in your building." If your practice grows rapidly, you will want this option to expand rather than relocate.

In Chapter 9 we described the basic pieces of furniture and equipment necessary to start up the medical practice. In the following pages, we will discuss the office telephone system and computer system.

Acquiring Equipment

Leasing Versus Purchasing

Leasing entails higher interest rates, but requires lower down payments. Before acquiring equipment items, discuss with your accountant the advantages of leasing versus purchasing. Generally, because of limited access to capital in a practice start-up, highly technical equipment should be leased rather than purchased. Most vendors will offer the option to lease equipment. Further, most leasing companies will offer several leasing options. After your purchase price is established, your accountant will calculate and advise you on the best way to attain the item, based on the capital you have available, current interest rates, the technology of the equipment, and the total cash investment requirements of your practice start-up.

Your Office Telephone System

The telephone is your primary connection to your patients. Choose a system that will fulfill your needs. It is not necessary that you purchase a system now that has all the "bells and whistles" available on the market. However, do choose a system that has the expansion capability you may need in the future.

The cost of a telephone system is based on the number of lines the main unit can accommodate. The smallest system is usually four lines. The next size would be six lines, then eight lines, etc. The plan should be to purchase a system that will accommodate the number of lines you need now plus two to four more lines for future expansion.

Plan for a line dedicated for a facsimile machine and another for a computer modem. You will need a minimum of four "hunting" lines, plus two dedicated lines, totaling six; eight is ideal to start. Expect to pay between $2,500 and $5,000 for a basic system with four to six lines. Consider the following information to assist you in making your final choice.

Before making any equipment purchase, check with your local telephone company to see what central office services are available. Your investment requirements may be reduced, or at least delayed, during the initial phase of your practice start-up by taking advantage of external services.

Determine Equipment Needs

Using the following list, decide what equipment you will need. Consider what features and services you want?

- Local telephone lines (e.g., inbound, outbound, dedicated, etc.)
- Intercom
- Hands-free capability
- Reception room phone (Make sure you block long distance access.)
- After-hours service
- Yellow Pages listing (Determine the publication date.)

Select Potential Vendors

There are two types of companies that provide telephone service and equipment. They are as follows:

- The local telephone company, who supplies and services telephone lines, telephone instruments, and related equipment.

- Interconnect companies, e.g., independent firms that provide and service telephone instruments and related equipment.

Use this list of resources to *obtain recommendations* and check references for vendors in your area:

- Colleagues, other business users

- Local medical societies

- Hospitals

- Credit bureaus

- Better Business Bureau

- Others

Compare costs by obtaining quotations on equipment and service; be sure all costs are included and separately designated. For example:

- Purchase costs

- Termination fees, if leasing

- Federal, state and local taxes

- Shipping charges

- Installation fees

- "Cut-over" charges (usually a part of the installation fee)

- Warranty

- Post warranty maintenance charges

- Interest (for installment purchases)

- Capacity for expansion; plan for your future.

Compare the extras offered by each vendor:

- Peak load study

- Busy signal study

- Training programs

It is easy to over buy telephone service and equipment. Of primary importance is that you purchase wisely, selecting equipment that is easy to upgrade as your practice needs grow.

The Office Computer System

Whatever the size of your practice, you will benefit by having an automated office. In this age of computer technology, beginning your practice without a computer is pointless. Computer systems are much like telephone systems; the more features they have, the more they cost. The computer hardware is only a small portion of the system's cost. The practice management software you purchase will be a larger and more important expenditure.

Computerized systems offer many benefits to a solo, small, and medium-sized medical practices. They can be used for the following purposes:

- Improve the quality of patient records, billing and other office procedures.

- Reduce accounts receivable and increase cash flow because of reduced claims submission errors and delays.

- Assemble and display data on your fees, reimbursement percentage and collections percentage that will allow you to develop pricing strategies to improve your cash flow.

- Compile information on the characteristics of your patient population, your referral patterns, the average length of time your patients spend in the hospital, and the most common procedures you provide. This information can be used to develop marketing plans that will help you attract more patients and the attention of managed care organizations or group practices with which you would like to establish a relationship.

- Decrease the time required to enter the same data on several different forms (patient's record, accounting/billing system, medical records, etc.).

- Establish new office routines that might not be feasible in a manual system (e.g., sending thank-you notes to patients who refer friends or relatives, retrieving names of patients with similar diagnoses to remind them of the need for periodic checkups, etc.).

In selecting management software, choose a program that can perform these functions:

- *Billing, collecting, and insurance processing*
    - Accounts receivable
    - Aging analysis of accounts receivable
    - Standard collection form letters that can be personalized
    - Preparation of insurance claims
    - Direct claims data entry to insurance company
    - Patient billing (on demand and cyclical)
    - Reminder system for claims follow-up

- *Accounting*
    - Accounts payable
    - Annual statements to patients
    - Cash register
    - Check writing
    - Cross-posting in multi physician practices
    - Automatic day sheet and deposit slip
    - General ledger

- Income and expense statement
- Payroll and payroll records
- Profit and loss statements
- Retirement plan accounting
- Preparation of W-2, corporate and individual tax forms

■ *Practice Management*
- Patient profiles by age, diagnosis, procedure, service, home address, insurance carrier
- Productivity reports by physician (number of patients, gross revenue, supplies ordered, etc.)
- Referral profiles (patients and physicians)
- Employee vacation and absence records
- Lists of hospitalized patients and charges
- Linkage to satellite offices
- Inventories of drugs, supplies and equipment
- Automatic reminders of equipment and facilities maintenance needs
- Financial planning and modeling, practice analysis and research
- Business projections
- Analysis and correlation of patient data

■ *Scheduling and follow-up*
- Appointment scheduling and follow-up appointments
- Patient recall lists
- Patient reminders
- Daily printout of appointments scheduled

■ *Clinical Applications*
- Access to national data banks (including organ banks and burn registries) and reference works
- Continuing medical education programs
- Drug interaction and allergy checks
- Literature retrieval
- Medical records
- Patient and staff education
- Prescription writing
- Protocols, diagnosis and treatment
- Research

■ *Word Processing*
- Preparation of journal articles, patient newsletters, staff manuals, etc.
- Consultation reports
- Correspondence
- Labels, address lists, mail merges, etc.
- Thank you letters
- "Welcome to the practice" letters

In a managed care market, the physician who can control and retrieve patient data and clinical outcomes will be positioned best to negotiate fees with managed care organizations (MCOs). Your computer software should provide all the functions as listed above and have the following capabilities for evaluating managed care contracts:

- Measure financial performance and precise contractual allowance.

- Audit actual versus expected payment.

- Measure major employers and volume of business within each contract.

- Provide a database for contract-specific UR/UM requirements and denied days by payer.

- Track contract terms, renegotiation date, and reimbursement methodology.

- Track attending, admitting, referring physician and surgeon utilization and financial performance.

- Provide for repricing sheet or supplemental invoice.

- Allow for mixing multiple reimbursement methodologies and stop-loss provisions within the same contract.

- Link payer, employer and managed care party yet allow for multiple variations.

- Automatically link patient records to contracts. Calculate expected reimbursements and prorate amounts during importing or on demand for an individual patient record.

- Calculate late payment penalties that may eliminate negotiated discount or be based as additional interest.

- Provide tickler system for notification of expiring contracts.

- Identify key decision-makers for employers, payers and contracting entities.

- Allow for unlimited "carve-out" benefit combinations.

- Allow for multi institution multi contracts that may include two hospitals, ambulatory surgery center, home health and home infusion companies and physician practices.

- Track and audit secondary payer contracts.

- Allow for multiple reports with examples provided.

- Adequately handle physician- and hospital-specific reimbursement methodologies and contracts.

- Provide a relational database with open database connectivity (ODBC).

- Be user-friendly, flexible in use.

- Be available in multi user network version.

- Compare profit by patient, contract, DRG (or other payment methodology), service, physician.

- Interface with cost accounting application.

- Allow for "what if" pricing scenario by product line for per diem, per case, CPT-4 fee schedules, ICD-9 fee schedules, and compute outlier variations.

- Provide customized programs based on a practice case mix and charge data.

- Compare specific contract rates to practice contract averages and identify variances.

- Produce monthly and quarterly analysis reports by contract with volume of patients, payments, write-offs, revenue and expected reimbursement.

Electronic Medical Records (EMR)

While EMR are seldom found in medical practices today, this concept is the wave of the future. Many practice management software programs will allow an interface with an EMR module. Be sure that the practice management software you purchase will accommodate this interface in the future.

The purchase of a computer system will be your largest single expenditure. The initial expenditure required to purchase a reliable multi user system will be about $25,000. Attain expert advice before you purchase a system. A practice management consultant can assist you with your decision.

Contact several vendors and request a demonstration of their product. Get references from present clients, and if possible go to a location where the system is in use.

CHAPTER 11

Managing Personnel

Employment Law

A physician is viewed as an authority figure in a medical practice—even if he or she is also an employee. The clinical assistants and administrative staff expect the physicians to understand and follow the rules. If you plan to become an employee of a group practice, hospital or other entity, you should have a working knowledge of the laws and statutes regulating the medical practice, and a thorough understanding of the internal personnel guidelines that pertain to managing the employees.

All physicians should read this chapter. If you plan to open a private practice, you will need this basic information. You will also need to have more in-depth knowledge of your responsibilities under the law. Resources are furnished at the end of this chapter that will give the physician/ employer extensive information concerning employment law.

Civil Rights Act of 1964, Title VII

Commonly called Title VII, a brief description of this statute is as follows:

- Covers all employers with 15 or more employees who work 20 or more hours per week.

- Prohibits employment discrimination based on race, sex, religion, national origin or color.

- Prohibits retaliation against anyone seeking to enforce their rights.

- Established the Equal Employment Opportunity Commission (EEOC) to serve as an enforcement agency for Title VII.

Title VII has several amendments.

> **Pregnancy Discrimination Act of 1978.** An amendment to Title VII, this legislation makes it unlawful to discriminate on the basis of pregnancy.

> **Sexual Harassment.** Sexual harassment includes, but is not limited to, unwelcome sexual advances, request for sexual favors, and other verbal or physical conduct of a sexual nature. These definitions are intentionally broad and should prompt the employer to have specific policies in place that strictly prohibit any action that could be construed as sexual harassment.

Federal Age Discrimination in Employment Act of 1967 (ADEA)

This legislation makes it is unlawful for an employer to discipline or discharge an employee who is over 40 because of the employee's age. The ADEA does not regulate job-related discipline.

Americans with Disabilities Act of 1990

The ADA protects disabled persons from discrimination in employment, public services, public accommodations and telecommunications. The ADA has two components that affect the employer. The first one pertains to discrimination in hiring or employment and requires an employer to make reasonable accommodations for a disabled employee if they can perform the essential functions of the job. The second component pertains to accommodations that must be provided in order for disabled persons to access your facility or services. These accommodations for example, would include having a wheelchair ramp or a restroom that is large enough to accommodate a wheelchair.

The Fair Labor Standards Act of 1938 (FLSA)

Administered by the Department of Labor, a brief overview of this legislation is as follows:

- Established minimum wage.
- Regulates child labor.
- Establishes overtime pay.

The FLSA requires that employers keep records on wages and hours worked. You must be able to prove the number of hours an employee works each week. The Department of Labor does not require a special format for wage records as long as the required information is easily ascertainable. Wage records should include the following:

- The employee's full name as used in Social Security Administration records.
- The employee's Social Security Number, employee number or symbol, as used in payroll records.
- The employee's home address, including ZIP code.
- The employee's date of birth if the employee is under the age of 19.
- The employee's sex.
- The employee's position title.
- The time of the day and the day of the week the employee's work begins.
- The regular hourly rate of pay.
- The amount and type of pay for any pay that is not included in the "regular rate."
- The hours worked by the employee on each work day, and the total hours worked for the week.
- The employee's total daily or weekly earnings (not including any premiums paid for overtime).
- The employee's total payment of overtime for the work week.
- Total wages for the employee for each pay period.
- The date of each payment made to the employee and the pay period covered by the payment.
- The total amount of additions to or deductions from wages for each pay period.

- For each deduction, the employer must show the following:
  - date
  - amount
  - nature of the deduction

Unless the employee is exempt from overtime pay, the employer must pay one and one-half times the employee's regular rate of pay for all time worked over 40 hours in one work week. Even if an employer pays every two weeks, there can be no "averaging" of hours in the pay period. If the employee works 30 hours the first week of the pay period and 50 hours the next week, he or she is entitled to 10 hours overtime pay for the second week. Overtime is based on hours **worked** over 40, not including vacation and sick leave taken during the same pay period.

Employment Categories

The administrator should become familiar with the laws governing work hours and wage payments, including minimum wages, overtime, deductions from wage, and child labor. Refer to the Fair Labor Standards Act (FLSA) to obtain a working knowledge of this national policy on minimum wages and overtime payments. This complex law determines whether an employer is subject to federal minimum wage and overtime requirements. Most medical employees are covered. First, ascertain the status of your practice. Then, conclude the exempt or nonexempt status of each employee.

Exempt. The following employment categories have been adapted for application to the medical practice for defining employees who are exempt from overtime pay requirements.

- An *Executive Employee* must meet all of the following definitions to be exempt: (Practice Administrators are typically considered exempt.)
  - Primary duty consists of the management of the practice or a customarily recognized department.
  - Must supervise at least two full-time employees.
  - Must have authority to hire and fire or to recommend those actions.
  - Must regularly exercise discretionary powers.
  - Must spend no more than 20 percent of working hours on nonmanagerial duties.

- An *Administrative Employee* must meet the following definitions to be exempt (administrative assistants, personnel directors, office managers, and laboratory supervisors are typically considered exempt):
  - Primary duty must be responsible office or nonmanual work directly related to management policy or general business operations.
  - Must regularly exercise discretion and independent judgment.
  - Must have authority to make important decisions.
  - Must assist the executive.
  - Must not spend more than 20 percent of work week in non-administrative duties.

- A *Professional Employee* must meet all the following requirements to be exempt (physicians, registered nurses, registered or certified medical technologists, physician assistants, speech pathologists, and physical therapists are typically considered exempt):
  - Primary duty must be work requiring knowledge of an advanced type in a field of science, usually obtained by a prolonged course of specialized instruction and study.
  - Must consistently exercise discretion and judgment.

– Must do work that is mainly intellectual and varied.

– Must not spend more than 20 percent of work week on activities not a part of or incident to professional duties.

Nonexempt. Among common positions that typically are considered *nonexempt* are the following:

- Licensed practical nurses.

- Nurses' aides.

- Laboratory technicians or assistants.

- Clerical workers.

- Orderlies.

- Food service employees.

- Janitorial employees.

At-Will Contracts

The most common type of employment agreement in the health care industry is the oral, "at-will" agreement. This establishes a relationship in which the employer and employee work at the will of the other. Understanding this relationship is important.

Concept: Just as an employee can quit at any time, so can the employer terminate the employee at any time, with or without reason.

Exceptions: "At-will" does not apply to a job in which a contract is in effect stating a specific period of employment. The right of the employer to apply the "at-will" doctrine does not override the restrictions placed on the employer such as the discriminations defined in Title VII of the 1964 Civil Rights Act.

By using the term "at-will" versus "just cause," an employee serves at the discretion of the medical practice and therefore may be dismissed with or without cause. Utilization of the term "just cause" sets a prerequisite that justifiable cause must be shown in order to discharge an employee. Use specific language in your employee handbook (discussed later in this chapter) to indicate that employees of your practice are employees "at will."

Posting Requirements

Federal and state laws often require employers to post a notice about a particular law. These notices are usually provided as posters or permits and should be placed in a conspicuous place easily accessible to all employees (i.e., the break room). Listed below are the posters that employers are required to display under federal law. Not all are required of every employer. Refer to the specifications listed previously in this chapter to see if your practice qualifies.

Age Discrimination, Disability Discrimination, Equal Employment

- Poster titled "Equal Employment Opportunity Is the Law."

- Available from EEOC offices.

Child Labor, Minimum Wage and Overtime

- Wage-hour poster 1088 (Federal Minimum Wage).
- Available from the U.S. Department of Labor.

Family and Medical Leave

- Poster required by Family and Medical Leave Act of 1993.
- Available from the U.S. Department of Labor.

Polygraph Testing

- Wage-hour poster 1462 (Employee Polygraph Protection Act) required.
- Available from the U.S. Department of Labor.

Safety

- OSHA poster 2203 (Job Safety & Health Protection) required.
- Available from the U.S. Department of Labor.
- OSHA also requires posting an annual summary of on-the-job injuries (OSHA Form 200).

The posters may be obtained from the government agency charged with enforcing a particular law. Most agencies have developed a single poster that satisfies the requirements of several different laws administered by that agency. There are also private companies that publish posters that employers are required to have. Contact the following agencies to obtain these posters:

Equal Employment Opportunity Poster Office
2401 E. Street N.W.
Washington, D.C. 20507

U. S. Department of Labor Posters
200 Constitution Ave. N.W., Room S-3502
Washington, D.C. 20210

Workers' Compensation

Physicians usually think of Workers' Compensation only regarding the medical care it provides to other employers' workers. However, the physician is an employer as well and must cover his own employees with Workers' Compensation Insurance.

State law governs Workers' Compensation almost entirely. The majority of employers are insured through private carriers. Most states require that employers comply with the Workers' Compensation Law in one of two ways:

- purchasing Workers' Compensation insurance through a qualified carrier or a state insurance fund
- becoming self-insured by a process prescribed by state law.

You can receive information that outlines your responsibilities by contacting the Workers' Compensation Board in your state. They will provide you with a packet of information for the new employer. Your insurance agent is also a good resource for information about Workers' Compensation requirements.

OSHA Workplace Requirements

The Occupational Safety and Health Administration (OSHA) was enacted in 1970 to assure safe, healthful working conditions for employees. Employers are required to furnish employees a place of employment that is safe from recognized hazards. In the medical office the hazards of greatest concern are "blood borne pathogens."

It is the responsibility of every medical employer to obtain complete information for compliance with OSHA regulations. The OSHA Handbook for Small Businesses, which includes self-inspection checklists, is available from local OSHA offices.

Hiring Employees

All employees need guidelines and rules to understand what is expected of them. A well-written job description is the best way of communicating a description of the duties for which an employee is responsible.

Your priority should be to hire an experienced office manager. Expect to pay a higher wage to an experienced person, but by doing so you will recoup this extra expenditure in efficiency and dollars collected. Once your front office person has been hired, he or she can develop job descriptions and screen applicants for your clinical assistant.

Give a great deal of thought to the duties of the office manager and prepare a job description before you begin the advertising or hiring process. A job description usually includes the following elements:

Job Title. The name of the job.

Job Summary. A one- or two-sentence summary that defines the overall function of the job.

Job Qualifications. A brief listing of educational and experience qualifications

Duties and Responsibilities. A list of the major job tasks describing what is to be accomplished.

Sample job descriptions for an office manager and a clinical assistant are provided at the end of this chapter.

Setting a Salary Range

Personnel salaries and benefits will be your largest single expense. You will want to hire the person with the best skills for what you can afford to pay. Developing a salary range for each job title is the recommended way to set salaries. Staff salaries should be predicated on the following:

- How much the practice can afford to pay now and what you what you can probably pay next year.

- The average salary for the same job within the community for staff with the same level of experience and education.

Before comparing salaries with other offices, make sure you compare the job description as well.

Sources for Developing a Pool of Candidates

- Office Managers' Professional Associations
- Community Colleges
- Private Vocational Schools
- Local Chapters of Health Care Organizations, such as the American Association of Medical Assistants.
- Medical Societies' Placement Service
- Pharmaceutical Representatives
- Hospital Personnel Department
- Employment Agencies

Placing an Effective Classified Advertisement

The Civil Rights Act of 1964 (Title VII) also applies to the advertising, application and hiring process. Ads must be carefully written to avoid any appearance of discrimination based on gender, age, race, religion, national origin or disability. Use the basic components of the job description to formulate your ad. Focus on what the job requires rather than the type of person you prefer. When placing a newspaper advertisement, have candidates send their written resumes to a box number rather than listing a telephone number or your office address.

Preparing for the Interview

Review the written resumes you have received and choose at least five candidates you feel have the qualifications you require. Give each of these resumes a priority rating. Screen your top five applicants by phone first. You may choose to have all five come in for a face-to-face interview, or you can narrow your choices to two or three candidates.

Be organized in the face-to-face interviews, having a list of questions prepared to ask each candidate. This will allow you to compare the candidates on the same basis. Give each interviewee a copy of the job description and have him complete an EEOC (Equal Employment Opportunity Commission)-approved application form. Using an EEOC form will assure that you are not violating any of the Title IV statutes. These forms are available through the American Medical Association Publications Department, office supply stores, and most mail order catalogs offering forms for the medical office. An example appears at the end of this chapter.

Every employer develops his or her own interviewing style. You may want to begin your interviews by telling the candidate a little about yourself or your practice. Share with the candidate why you chose that particular geographic area, where you went to school and what is your philosophy about the practice of medicine. Next you may wish to proceed in the following manner:

- Ask the candidate if he has reviewed the job description and whether he has any questions about the essential functions of the job.

- Ask each applicant about his experience with each task listed on the job description. Ask how he performs these tasks in his current position or in former jobs. Write the answers on a separate piece of paper. Do not write on the job description, application form or resume.

- Ask open-ended questions that will require the applicant to provide information. Avoid questions that can be answered yes or no.

- Remain neutral in your responses. Do not show approval or disapproval.
- Watch for nonverbal clues that indicate tension or anxiety.
- Zero in on subjects of interest to you and investigate further.
- Quickly review your objectives.
- Document key points
- Let the candidate know what happens next.

Interviewing Questions

Use this list of questions with each candidate making notes on a separate paper, not on the resume of application.

- What did you like best about your last (current) position? What did you like least about it?
- Which of your past positions did you find most satisfying? Why?
- How would your last (current) supervisor describe you? In what area would he say you need the most improvement?
- What is one of your most significant on-the-job accomplishments?
- What academic areas of study interest you the most? What, if any, helped prepare you for your field?
- What did you like best about your last supervisor? What did you like least?
- What change would you (or did you) make in the last office you worked in?
- Describe your experiences in collecting money for medical bills.
- Which of your skills do you think you could develop here?

Checking References

Reference checking is vitally important to the medical employer. Previous employers are generally reluctant to convey information on employees. However, using finesse and gentle persuasion, you can usually obtain the information you need to make a hiring decision. Be sure to thank the person with whom you speak for their cooperation.

- Request that each applicant provide you with two or three references. A former employer or supervisor is preferred.
- Call the references instead of accepting "letters of reference."
- Ask to speak to the applicant's immediate supervisor.
- Ask if the applicant is eligible for rehiring.
- Listen for what they do not say.

The Probationary Period

When hiring, inform the new employee that he will be subject to a ninety-day probationary period. Use this time for orientation and training. During this period, monitor the employee's attitude, work habits and capabilities and assure that he is receiving the proper instructions.

The employee or the employer may end the employment relationship "at-will" at any time during this probationary period, with or without cause, and without advance notice. Employees will assume "regular" status upon satisfactory completion of the probationary period.

On the first day, present the employee with a copy of the Employee Handbook or Personnel Manual. Take time to explain the basic work rules and regulations including:

- Compensation and benefits
- Payroll deductions
- Vacation schedules and sick leaves
- Safety and health

Help the employee have a global view of the practice and see how his job fits into the overall plan. This explanation will emphasize the importance of the new employee s role and will encourage pride in the job and the practice.

Ask the employee to read the manual. Offer to answer any questions about policy and procedures. Address any tentative issues such as dress codes, overtime, etc. *After they have reviewed the manual, the employee should sign an acknowledgment form. Place a copy of the acknowledgment form in the personnel file.*

Setting Up the Personnel File

Every employee, including the physicians, should have a personnel file. Each file should contain the documents listed below and be maintained appropriately.

Personnel File Contents. The typical file should contain all government-mandated forms and employee benefit enrollment forms, as applicable:

- Resumé
- Employment Application
- Reference Checklist
- W-4 Form
- State Income Tax Form, if applicable
- Form I-9
- Payroll Set-Up Information
- Health Insurance Enrollment Form
- Long-Term Disability Enrollment Form
- 401(k) Enrollment Form
- Flex Benefits Form
- Personnel Policies Acknowledgment Form (Disclaimer)
- Attendance Records
- Employment Letter
- Salary Change Information
- Performance Reviews

- Warning or Disciplinary Letters
- New Employee Checklist
- Training Checklist
- Confidentiality Pledge
- Contact list in case of an emergency

Employer Access and Retention. Personnel files should be kept in a locked cabinet, accessible only to the designated employee responsible for their maintenance.

Employee Access. The employee has the right to access his file at any time, in the presence of a designated employee.

Retention. An employee's personnel file should be retained for three years following termination. Applications of persons not hired should be maintained for one year.

Performance Appraisals and Salary Review

Each employee should have a performance appraisal every year. This appraisal is usually conducted on the anniversary of the employee's hire date. The following list gives some pointers on conducting a successful performance review:

- Use a preprinted form. Give the employee a copy a week or two in advance and ask him to evaluate his own performance.

- Do not conduct a salary review when you are reviewing performance. If you combine the two, employees will concentrate on dollars rather than performance.

- Allow an adequate amount of time. Avoid rushing through!

- Conduct the appraisal in a confidential atmosphere.

- Set specific goals and time lines for improvement.

- Close the discussion with a compliment.

Salary Reviews

As a matter of necessity, salary increases must be based on practice profits. When funds are available to give employees a salary increase, it should be based on merit. Based on an employee's performance, merit raises can be motivators in that they recognize special effort or provide an incentive to improve. Know who is contributing what and how much. Do not be afraid to make a distinction; this is the point of merit raises.

Make sure your employees understand how salary increases are calculated and how they are given. Explain the process in your Employee Handbook.

Counseling, Discipline and Termination

Managing a staff requires counseling, discipline, and some eventual terminations. Make every effort to work with your employees to help them give their best to their duties. Note and file in the personnel file any disciplinary discussions held with the employee, documenting what was said and the subsequent response. These records will substantiate the reasons for termination, if this action becomes necessary. Having proper documentation reduces your exposure to loss from claims brought by a disgruntled employee.

Before beginning the termination process, keep the following points in mind:

- Often, potential grounds for dismissal are present at the time an employee is hired. Be sure you check all past references thoroughly and have an understanding of how the applicant got along with previous coworkers, supervisors, and patients.

- Employees must understand the terms of any probationary period. It is important they know the grounds for dismissal, that no advance notice will be given, that severance pay and unemployment benefits may not be extended. (Check your state statues.)

- All policies governing grounds for dismissal, disciplinary procedures, grievance procedures, etc., must be clearly outlined in your personnel manual. Be sure that you apply your standards equally and impartially to all.

- Any decision to terminate should be the final step in a clearly documented and well-defined process. Make sure you have exhausted all alternatives first.

There may be a host of reasons why you have decided to begin the disciplinary process for an employee, to explore other alternatives to termination. The employee must be made aware of unsatisfactory performance or behavior and be given a chance to improve; after giving ample opportunity to no avail, you should terminate the employee without delay.

The Employee Handbook

A key part of an employer's communication program is the Employee Handbook. It provides information on basic rules and policies that affect job conditions and should be issued when an employee begins employment. The following general information is to help you decide what to include in a handbook. Your staff needs to understand:

- What you expect of them and what they can expect of you.

- Your policies on wages, working conditions, and benefits.

- What services your practice provides to patients.

The Employee Handbook should reflect the mission and philosophy of the physician. Handbooks protect the employer. Guesswork can be eliminated when either the employer or employee can refer to a written policy.

Handbooks give employees a sense of security. With all the rules and policies in one place, each person knows what is expected of him. When benefits are listed and explained, each person knows what is provided. Handbooks can also help motivate employees.

The Format—How You Want It to Look

Choose a size for your handbook that is easy to use. Typical sizes are 3-1/2" X 6-1/2" or 5" X 7". Books can be loose-leaf or bound. Bound books are less expensive than loose-leaf, but loose-leaf notebooks allow for replacement of pages when policies change. Some employers use both formats—a small bound "handbook" for employees, and a loose-leaf policy and procedures manual for managers. Both books should include an employee acknowledgment form.

Make your booklet attractive; put it together in such as way that employees will want to read it. Consider these suggestions for making the contents easy to read:

- Limit the use of words with three or more syllables.
- Keep each sentence 20 words or less.
- Limit discussion of subjects to one page.
- Use drawings, charts, and cartoons where applicable.
- Leave at least one quarter of each page blank.
- Limit the number of pages

Choose a writing style and be consistent throughout. Use gender-neutral terminology. A handbook should cover what employees need to know to get along on the job the policies and procedures that employees will encounter almost every day. Avoid subjects that change frequently, such as a lengthy and detailed descriptions of benefits plans.

The following sample table of contents can be used as a checklist for deciding what to include in a handbook.

Sample Table of Contents

Welcome Letter and Introduction
- Letter of Appreciation to Current Employees
- Letter of Welcome to New Employees
- Purpose of Handbook
- Background of Practice
    - Organization Chart
    - Physician(s)' Biographical Information
- Equal Employment Opportunity Statement
- Suggestion and Complaint Procedures

Employment Policies and Procedures
- Nature of Employment
- Probationary Period
- Employment Relations
- Supervisor's Responsibilities
- Employee's Role and Responsibilities
- Work Schedules
- Rest and Meal Periods
- Overtime Policy
- Attendance and Punctuality
- Time Cards
- Personnel Records
- Payday
- Payroll Deductions
- Performance and Salary Review
- Resignation/Termination
- Telephone Use

Benefits
- Holidays
- Vacations
- Hospital and Medical Insurance
- Life Insurance
- Pension and Profit-Sharing
- Training
- Educational Assistance Program
- Service Awards
- Workers' Compensation
- Sick Leave
- Disability Leave
- Personal Leave
- Bereavement Leave
- Jury Duty
- Witness Duty

Safety
- Safety Rules
- Emergency Procedures
- Personal Protective Equipment
- Reporting Accidents

Employee Conduct and Disciplinary Action
- Standards of Conduct
- Confidentiality Policy
- Smoking Policy
- Drug, Alcohol and Substance Abuse Policy (Including testing, if applicable)
- Sexual and Other Forms of Impermissible Harassment
- Security Inspections
- Solicitation
- Personal Appearance and Dress Code
- Corrective Discipline Procedures

Summary and Acknowledgment
- Disclaimer Statement

Keep in mind that employee handbooks vary considerably due to individual needs and circumstances; therefore, the amount of information provided varies. A medical practice may also consider publishing OSHA, CLIA and other government-regulated topics in its handbook. For the overall purpose of a handbook, mentioning these rules in passing would be most appropriate, while covering them more extensively in other documentation (i.e., Policy Manual). If this is done, be sure your acknowledgment form covers all policies.

Sample Job Descriptions

The following job descriptions are provided as samples of positions in a medical practice. Use these examples for preparing your specific descriptions as required in your practice. Also use job descriptions for performance appraisals and for counseling employees. As responsibilities change, revise the descriptions accordingly.

Job Description

Position: Office Manager

Reports To: Physician(s)

Job Summary: Responsible for all medical office activities, including accounting and financial procedures. Supervise all office personnel.

Specific Requirements:

- Furnish physician, accountant with account aging each month.
- Conduct regular staff meetings.
- Responsible for accounts payable system.
- Supervise, train all front office personnel.
- Assist in creating, updating business administration policies.
- Update office personnel policy manual as needed.
- Maintain controls on accounts receivable system.
- Prepare financial reports at end of month for physician, accountant.
- Approve all Medicaid, Medicare and other write-offs in consultation with physician.
- Approve credits, refunds to patient accounts.
- Arrange personnel schedules and vacations.
- Responsible for all hiring and terminating of office personnel.
- Conduct performance, salary reviews for office personnel.

Job Qualifications:

BA or AA degree in Business Administration required. Previous medical office experience also required. Supervisory experience preferred. Knowledge of medicolegal principles and medical ethics necessary.

Job Description

Position: Medical Assistant—Clinical

Reports To: Office Manager

Job Summary: Assist physician with patient examination and treatment. Also responsible for patient histories, routine lab procedures, collection and preparation of specimens for transport to lab.

Specific Requirements:

- Maintain general appearance, cleanliness of exam rooms.

- Sterilize instruments, maintain diagnostic equipment.

- Prepare, replenish supplies. Maintain inventory.

- Prepare, drape patients for examination.

- Take patient histories, height, weight, temperature.

- Give certain medications, injections under physician supervision.

- Assist in collection of specimens. Instruct patients regarding preparation for tests.

- Record laboratory, x-ray, EKG data on patient charts.

- Receive and organize the handling of medication samples.

- Dispose of contaminated and disposable items.

- Perform other tasks as requested by office manager or physician.

Job Qualifications:

Graduate of medical assisting course or nursing program. Previous clinical experience and knowledge of anatomy, physiology and terminology also required. Medical office experience helpful.

CHAPTER 12

Developing Policies and Procedures

Developing a Policies and Procedures Manual

Every medical practice should have written policies and procedures. A well-written Policies and Procedures Manual will provide a training and orientation guide for new employees, and serve as an ongoing reference for the office staff.

The Policies and Procedures Manual should be prepared with greater detail and bound separately from the Employee Handbook. Each employee should sign a form acknowledging that he has read the practice policies. This form is maintained in the employee's personnel file.

The Policies and Procedures Manual should accomplish the following:

- Provide step-by-step guidelines for completion of each task in the office.

- Identify key personnel to use as resources for each task.

- Include samples of forms to be used.

- List frequently called telephone numbers.

- Advise about miscellaneous office matters (e.g., location of keys, how to reorder forms, etc.)

Specific policies and instructions should address the following functions:

- Communicating hospital and surgery charges

- Purchasing protocols

- Office collections routine

- Releasing patient records prerequisites

- Billing policies and follow up

- Registering a patient

- Setting up a patient's file

- Completing a superbill

- Scheduling patient appointments

- Closing and reconciling day's activities

- Cleaning laboratory equipment

- Performing an EKG

- Scheduling a laboratory test

- Handling laboratory results, e.g., notifying the patient, physician's responsibilities, etc.

The physician must assume responsibility for the preparation of the Policies and Procedures Manual in the early stages. You will want to define how you want each policy or procedure to be carried out or conducted. After the initial set up phase, you can probably turn this task over to your administrative staff for updates and maintenance. An example of an appointment scheduling policy follows at the end of the chapter. Use it as a format for writing your specific manual.

Types of Appointment Schedules

Inefficient patient scheduling can significantly impede the progress of your day. There are many effective methods from which to choose. Experiment with different appointment schedules to learn what works best for you.

The typical format: One patient is scheduled every 15 minutes with an extra 15 minutes allowed for complete physicals or new patients.

The wave method: Three patients are scheduled to arrive on the hour and half-hour. This type of scheduling is based on the concept that one patient will always be early, another on time and the third five to ten minutes late. Scheduling in waves assures that you will always have a patient ready to be seen. Even new patients and physical exams can be handled in this way since they will generally need lab work, EKG or some other ancillary service that will allow you time to see another patient.

Scheduling based on needs: Patients for follow-up visits or minor illnesses are scheduled back-to-back. New patients, procedures or physicals are scheduled as the first and last patient each morning and each afternoon.

Whatever method you use, let your office staff know that it is imperative that they make you aware if patients are waiting longer than 15 minutes. The staff should also be responsible for keeping the patients informed of any delays. Patients usually do not mind waiting an extra few minutes if they are updated on a regular basis and given the opportunity to reschedule.

Your own responsibility for your appointment schedule cannot be overstated. Being kept waiting is still the number one complaint of most patients. Patient satisfaction is crucial in today's managed care market, and being on time goes a long way toward achieving patient satisfaction.

Tips for Efficient Scheduling

Consider the following pointers when addressing scheduling issues. These tips will improve access and increase efficiencies, benefiting you and your patients. Ensure that your staff has this information available to them through your policies and procedures manual.

- Arrange office hours to fit community needs. Some doctors hold evening hours two or three times a week or Saturday morning for the convenience of their patients.

- Use an appointment book or form that you design yourself. In a partnership or group, the system should provide columns or color-coded books for each doctor. Provision must be made for evening and weekend coverage and vacations.

- Establish an office policy for screening phone calls. Be sure to set aside specific times for callbacks.

- When an emergency delays the doctor, explain the situation to waiting patients; give them a choice of waiting or of rescheduling. Patients not yet in the office should be contacted.

- When a patient requests an appointment time that is already filled, the receptionist should volunteer at least two other times that are available. Chances are that the patient will choose one of those offered.

- Identify your more lengthy appointment types, and your "high risk, no show" patients (i.e., new patients) and send them written or oral reminders.

- If canceling an appointment is necessary, notify the patient as soon as possible.

- If you make house calls or visits to other institutions, schedule these trips realistically so they do not conflict with office hours.

- Do not overcrowd the schedule. Allow two or three "breathers" during the day for catching up, work-ins or emergencies.

- On slow days, consider keeping a "stand by" list available of patients who can be called in on short notice in case of cancellations.

Sample Policy—Appointment Scheduling

ABC Medical Practice Policies and Procedures Manual
Appointment Scheduling

I. When the doctor is in the office and is running more than ___ minutes late:

   A. Explanation to patients already in reception area and those arriving:
       Suggest opportunity to reschedule?   ❏ Yes   ❏ No
   B. Call patients not yet at office?   ❏ Yes   ❏ No
       Suggest opportunity to reschedule?   ❏ Yes   ❏ No

II. When the doctor is in the office and is running more than ___ minutes late:

   A. Explanation to patients already in reception area and those arriving:
       Suggest opportunity to reschedule?   ❏ Yes   ❏ No

III. If doctor is delayed at hospital, ER, nursing home, etc.:

   A. Explanation to patients already in reception area and those arriving:
       Suggest opportunity to reschedule?   ❏ Yes   ❏ No
   B. Call patients not yet at office?   ❏ Yes   ❏ No
       Suggest opportunity to reschedule?   ❏ Yes   ❏ No

IV. Patients calling to cancel appointments should be asked the following questions:

_____

_____

_____

Be sure to document in chart and appointment book.

Call patients on "early call-in" those scheduled later in the week who might like to come in earlier.

V. Instructions/statements to callers who have previously been a "no-show":

_____

VI. Instructions/statements to patients being "worked-in":

_____

_____

VII. Office policy on non-emergency "drop-ins":

_____

_____

_____

VIII. Policy to follow when more than one family member hopes to be seen in an appointment time reserved for just one:

_____

_____

IX. Office policy for patients arriving more than ___ minutes late:

_____

_____

X. Office policy for patients arriving early:

_____

_____

XI. Office policy to follow when detail people arrive without an appointment:

_____

_____

CHAPTER 13

Billing and Reimbursement Protocols

Collecting at the Time of Service

The best opportunity you have to collect your fee is to ask the patient to pay while he is still in your office. Make sure you have a designated person assigned the responsibility of requesting payment for services. Having the right person in this role is critical to the collection process. This individual must be pleasant, mature and well trained. Following these simple and practical rules will increase the probability of collecting payment at the time of service.

Do's and Don'ts. Use collection etiquette or "good manners" when collecting from a patient by remembering these pointers:

- DO respect the patient's privacy.
- DO use eye contact.
- DO address the patient by name.
- DON'T ask if the patient would like to pay.
- DO be prepared to explain the services and charges.
- DO be prepared to offer payment options if the patient is unable to pay in full.
- DON'T confront the patient.
- DON'T humiliate or embarrass the patient.
- DO smile and say "Thank you!"

Initial or Return Visit. When patients return, routinely follow these steps:

- Address the patient by name.
- Itemize the fees.
- Ask for payment.
- Provide payment options.
- Remember to say "Thank you!"

Previous Balance or Partial Payment. Use a polite, matter-of-fact attitude to approach a patient about a previous balance. Follow these steps to maximize your opportunity to collect:

- Address the patient by name.
- Itemize the fees for today's visit.

- Remind the patient of his previous balance.
- If they make partial payment, set up (and record) a payment agreement.
- Offer the patient a payment envelope.
- Remember to say "Thank you!"

Interfacing With Insurance Companies

Between 80 and 90 percent of your patients are covered by some form of insurance. An efficient computer system will take most of the "hassles" out of claims processing. However, the more you know about how insurance companies work, the more successful you will be in collecting your reimbursements. Following are descriptions of various plans and coverages you will encounter as you render medical services to patients.

Indemnity Plans

The traditional insurance companies are known as indemnity or commercial insurance plans. Sometimes called 80/20 plans, their marketing materials typically state that they pay 80 percent of the patient's medical bill, and the patient only pays the remaining 20 percent after an annual deductible is met. This type of advertising is misleading to the patient, because these companies base the 80 percent they pay on what they term a "usual and customary reimbursement" or UCR. The insurance company's UCR for a particular service is seldom, if ever, the same as your fee for that same service. Insurance companies generally do not explain how they establish their usual and customary fees.

Example:

You charge a patient $1,000 for repair of an inguinal hernia. The indemnity insurance plan says the usual and customary fee is $800, so they pay 80 percent of $800, not 80 percent of $1,000. The patient then is responsible for paying $360 to the physician instead of the $200 (or 20 percent of $1,000) they expected to pay. Often, the patient receives an explanation of benefits (EOB) that includes a statement similar to this: "Your physician's fee is higher than the usual and customary fee for this service/procedure. The usual and customary fee for this procedure is $800, so we are reimbursing 80 percent of $800."

The patient does not understand how the insurance company pays for a particular procedure, nor how this fee is calculated. Therefore, he becomes annoyed with the physician. Conducting some patient education before performing a service or surgical procedure is wise. Explain to the patient that your fee for the service may not be the same as the insurance company's reimbursement. Also explain that your fees are set so that you can provide a high quality service, pay your expenses and remain competitive in the marketplace. These communications are what keep the patients happy and set a successful physician apart from his peers.

Managed Care Plans

New physicians entering the marketplace today have an advantage in that they "grew up" with the managed care concept. Physicians who have been in private practice for many years have had to learn a new payment process and modify the way they view patient care.

In most areas today, several types of plans are offered, and most insurers sell some type of "managed care." The plans generally pay the provider on a discounted fee for service or a capitated basis.

Discounted Fee-for-Service Plans

In a discounted fee-for-service plan, the payer/insurance plan negotiates with the physician for a discount off his regular fee for a particular service in exchange for the promise of a potential increase in patients. Generally, the physician receives no guarantee in the number of patients he will receive from the plan. These plans are typically called Preferred Provider Organizations (PPO), Point of Service Plans (POS), or Health Maintenance Organizations (HMO).

Capitated Plans

In a capitated arrangement the physician agrees to provide a specified list of services to each patient assigned to his or her practice for a set dollar amount each month. The insurer pays the physician this specified amount whether or not the physician sees the patient in the office. This capitated amount may range from $3 per patient to $15 per patient depending on the specialty and the services the physician is required to provide within the capitated amount. This is often termed a "risk-sharing" arrangement.

Example:

The physician has 100 patients assigned to his practice for which the insurer pays him a capitated fee of $15 per member/per month (pm/pm), or a total of $1,500. If the physician sees 20 of these patients in a month and these patients require a total of $1,800 worth of services, the physician has lost $300. However, if the physician sees only five of the 100 patients in a month and their services total $200, the physician has made a gross profit of $1,300. Seeing the risk involved in this arrangement is easy.

The preceding description is an oversimplification of how reimbursement works in a managed care market. It is intended to help you understand the different types of insurance plans that you will encounter in a private practice. Before accepting and/or signing any kind of agreement with a managed care organization, you should understand the complexities of the system. Also, have an attorney review any contract before you sign it.

Workers' Compensation Insurance

All employers must provide Workers' Compensation Insurance. This insurance covers the medical and disability expenses incurred by the worker from a job-related injury. Many states administer Workers' Compensation Insurance billing directly. In these states, the physician sends the claims directly to the state's agency. Other states require employers to contract with an insurance company for payment of work-related claims. In either case, benefits and payments are predetermined by legislation, based on the state and the company. Request a packet of information from your state Workers' Compensation Board in preparation for accepting patients with work-related injuries and before processing claims.

When accepting a patient for work-related injury, remember these guidelines:

- The employer should authorize the treatment before you see the patient.

- Having a written request for treatment from the employer is best.

- If a written request is not possible, call the employer for authorization. Use a simple *Telephone Consent* form to record the authorization.

- The employer must notify the insurance company of the injury. If they do not file this "first report of injury," it will *delay* the physician's reimbursement.

- Treat Workers' Compensation claims as any insurance claim, filed in the unpaid claim file, and followed up routinely.

- Your first claim form should reach the insurance company within ten days of first treatment, even if treatment is completed.

- Physicians cannot bill patients for treatment of work-related injuries.

Insurance Filing and Follow Up

Insurance claims processing consumes a large portion of administrative time. Setting up workable policies and systems initially will help assure that insurance reimbursement provides a steady flow of cash into the practice.

Most medical management software can print the HCFA 1500 insurance form used for filing a claim with Medicare and Medicaid. This form is used, as well, with indemnity insurance carriers and managed care plans. Automation makes the filing process virtually "painless" and allows the practice to submit claims on a daily basis, if wanted. However, the claim filing process is only one small part of the reimbursement process. Monitoring the filed claims and assuring that insurers are paying them quickly requires much more effort. Develop a claim filing protocol similar to the following example to streamline this process:

- File claims at least twice weekly; daily is preferable.

- Check all claims for accuracy and completeness of information before mailing. Most insurance companies promise a 30-day turnaround time for payments if they receive a "clean claim."

- Print out a Claims Pending Report daily; call the insurance carrier on all claims that they have not paid within 30 days of the filing date. If your computer cannot generate this report, enter filed claims on an insurance log. Enter the date, the patients name, the insurance company and the amount filed on the log sheet. Check the log sheets every day to determine which claims they have not paid in thirty days and follow up by telephone.

- Call the insurance companies to ask about an unpaid claim. Calling is more effective than simply refiling the claim. If the insurance company says it has not received the claim, then refiling will be necessary.

- Print out an aged accounts analysis *by insurance company* each month to learn which companies pay on time and which ones habitually exceed a 30-day turnaround time. (This is not a standard report on every system. Requesting that the system be set up to provide this report is worthwhile.)

- Call the plan administrator and request an explanation of the plan's poor payment habits. Most managed care contracts guarantee a 30-day reimbursement schedule if the claims are submitted in order. If you do not receive your payments as agreed, it may be a sign that the plan is in financial trouble. If the payment problems persist, you may wish to terminate the contract.

- Make contractual adjustments at the time they make the payment.

- Conduct a periodic review of Explanation of Benefits (EOBs). An EOB statement, similar to a check stub, accompanies every insurance payment. Compare the EOB with the filed claim to assure that the insurer is paying claims appropriately, without reductions or denials.

Follow-up is the key to satisfactory reimbursement. If you produce your insurance claims on a "file and forget" method, you may find yourself with a cash flow shortfall. Give employees a copy of your written policy. Make them accountable for following these routines.

Billing the Patient

Every patient is personally responsible to you, the physician, for the payment of medical services rendered to them, even if they have insurance. You are not obligated to file the patient's insurance claims unless you have a contract with the insurance company. These contracted agreements include Medicare, Medicaid and Managed Care Plans. Agreeing to file a patient's insurance and wait for the reimbursement is a service you provide to your patients. This service is important, and it is surely one you need to provide. However, make sure the patient understands that payment is ultimately his responsibility.

Establish a written financial policy that you can present to your patients before they receive treatment. This financial policy should explain to the patient your payment expectations, and your policy on filing insurance claims. The following is a list of important points to include in your written financial policy:

- A statement that payment for services is expected at the time of service unless arrangements are made prior to treatment.

- The office will file insurance claims for services rendered, but the patients are not relieved of responsibility for payment because they have insurance.

- Patients must pay any copay or deductible due before a surgical procedure is performed and at the time the service is rendered (i.e., for office visits, etc.).

- Statements are mailed every 30 days. Any balance left unpaid for 90 days will be turned over to a collection agency.

- Financial arrangements can be made for payment of bills that are more than $XXX (you choose your limit).

Statements sent to patients for services rendered should include the entire amount due, even if an insurance company will pay most of it. Many practice management programs will produce statements that show both the amount presumed covered by insurance and the portion for which the patient is responsible.

Patients should receive statements regularly for any outstanding amount. Your billing cycle can be set up in several ways. The traditional method is to send all statements at the end of each month. Other methods include sending statements twice monthly, one half on the 15th and one half on the 30th. The third method is to send some statements out each week according to letters of the alphabet. These last two billing methods spread the cash flow and the associated payment posting work more evenly throughout the month.

- Send each patient a statement of his bill no more than 30 days after the date of service.

- Call each patient who has an unpaid bill 45 days after the date of treatment. Ask these patients if a problem has prevented payment of the bill. Make notes of any comments made by the patient.

- If the patient says that he cannot pay the full amount of his bill, offer to set up a payment schedule.

- Send the second statement 60 days after the date of service.

- If they do not pay payment by the 75th day following the date of service, make another phone call to the patient requesting payment. Record any comments.

- The third statement should go out 90 days after the date of service.

- If they do not make payment by the 100th day, send a letter to the patient stating that unless payment is received in ten days, the account will be turned over to an outside collection agency.

- At 110 days, turn any unpaid accounts over to a collection agency. Send the patient a letter of withdrawal stating that you will no longer be able to provide medical treatment.

Officially terminating the patient/physician relationship is important when they do not meet financial obligations. The physician cannot refuse to treat an established patient who owes the practice money unless he has formally terminated the relationship. See Chapter 14, Loss Prevention/Risk Management for more information on patient termination.

As with insurance filing and billing, a structured process for patient billing and follow-up is the most important factor in achieving reimbursement.

Using a Collection Agency

Approximately 2 percent of patients do not pay their medical bills. After you have exhausted all your in-house collection techniques, you may elect to turn some accounts over to a collection agency.

Choose a collection agency carefully. The agency's collection methods reflect on your practice. Talk with other physicians or office managers to see which agency they are using. Ask if they are satisfied with the services they receive and what percentage of accounts turned over for collection are paid. Collection agencies typically show a collection success rate of less than 25 percent. Use the following checklist for selecting a credible collection agency.

- Is the agency a member of the American Collectors Association?

- Is the agency in total compliance with the Fair Debt Collection Practices Act?

- What percentage of their business is medical?

- How are the accounts broken down per collector?

- How many accounts per collector?

- Does the agency have a training program?

- Does the monthly collection summary show when they listed the account and how much was paid?

- What are the agency's hours?

- Will they work accounts between 6:00 p.m. and 9:00 p.m. when most patients are available?

- How quickly does your account get on the desk of a collector?

- What reports do they provide?

- Does the agency report non-payers to the Credit Bureau?

- How long will the agency work on an account before they deem it *uncollectible*?

- How much commission do they charge?

Besides the items listed above, several points should be considered:

- Get copies of all the letters the agency will send to your patients.

- Do not turn over accounts of less than $50.

- Make a note on the patient's ledger card that you have turned over the account.

- Never pay commission up front.

- Make sure you can recall your accounts anytime.

- Have a written agreement. Read the fine print.

- Do not allow the agency to litigate an account without your permission.

- Report changes in the collection status of an account to the agency.

- Keep a log of all accounts in collection. Enter the name, date turned over, amount due, amount the patient paid, and your *net back*.

- Use two agencies simultaneously so you can evaluate their efficiency.

- Establish a time limit on how long an agency is entitled to a percentage of amounts collected after an account is withdrawn.

Using Credit Cards to Enhance Collections

Acceptance of credit cards for payment of medical bills is routine in most offices today. This offers an excellent option for physicians because it brings funds into the practice immediately, and transfers the risk of nonpayment to the credit card company.

Almost every bank offers vendor/merchant accounts that will allow you to deposit your credit card payments into the bank for processing. Some credit card companies will transfer the funds to your bank electronically so that you have access to the money immediately.

Every bank sets its own service charge for processing credit card transactions. They generally base these service charges on a percentage of your overall deposits and range from 2 percent to 8 percent. The service charge is often negotiable. If you have no deposit history with the bank, your negotiating "clout" may not be very strong. If the bank accepts electronic transfers of your funds from the credit card companies, the service charge should be lower.

Your credit card merchant account does not have to be in the same bank as your checking account. However, you will find that it is more convenient, and you will generally receive favorable service charge rates from your own bank.

This is the process for establishing a credit card account:

- Visit the bank where you have your office account. Explain that you want to set up merchant accounts for acceptance of credit card deposits. Ask what their service charges are. (Do not accept their first offer; attempt to negotiate the lowest rate possible.)

- Once they establish your account, the bank will assign you a merchant number. The bank will typically give you the necessary materials for accepting credit cards such as charge slips, credit slips, deposit slips, etc. They will also provide you with the machine that allows you to obtain approval from the credit card companies and have the funds transferred to your account electronically. This process may vary; every bank's credit card department has established protocols for merchant accounts.

- Ask the bank representative if having a bank employee come to your office is possible to set up the electronic transmittal unit and explain to your staff how the credit card process works.

Controlling the accounts receivable process will assure that your practice is financially successful. Collecting monies due you is not a process that "runs by itself." The physician should take an interest in this process. Establish measurable goals and make employees accountable for responsibilities in the process.

CHAPTER 14

Loss Prevention/Risk Management

Risk Management in the Medical Office

A steady increase has occurred in the number of medical malpractice claims over the past ten years. One can generally attribute these lawsuits to the following causes:

- Scientific advances that enable cures for certain previously untreatable conditions but, simultaneously, carry inherent risks of undesirable results or side effects.

- "The Marcus Welby Syndrome," i.e., unrealistic expectations of what can be done. Many people still expect a cure for every ailment.

- Reduced communication between physician and patient and the subsequent breakdown of personal rapport.

- An increasingly lawsuit-oriented society that seeks to hold someone at fault for injuries or accidents that were previously considered misfortune.

Developing a Loss Prevention Program

Any effective program of loss prevention must emphasize risk management and quality assurance. The physician and administrator must set into action a plan to accomplish the following:

- Identify existing or potential patient care problems.

- Establish criteria for patient care responsibility.

- Measure and monitor the actual performance of the staff.

- Investigate and resolve problems or complaints.

- Monitor the corrective action.

- Educate employees about government regulatory programs and the record keeping requirements for each program.

- Provide continuing education for both employees and patients.

The following subtitles address each area of practice operation individually and provide suggestions for developing a loss prevention protocol in these areas.

Scheduling

A common source of patient dissatisfaction in a physician's office is the length of time the patient must wait once he arrives for the appointment. When they endure long waits, patients perceive a lack of concern. A dissatisfied patient increases the risk of a professional liability claim. Consider these points when scheduling patients:

- The length of time it takes to get an appointment.

- The receptionist's demeanor.

- Whether the receptionist asks patients calling for an appointment permission before putting them on hold.

- The average length of time a patient is left on hold on the telephone.

The maximum time a patient should wait in the reception area is thirty minutes. If the wait is any longer, he becomes dissatisfied. To decrease the patient's wait time, follow these recommendations:

- Schedule extra time for new patients or special procedures.

- Allow enough time before and after seeing patients. Avoid over-booking patients.

- Inform patients of any delays in the appointment schedule and the cause for the delay.

- Call patients at home to advise them of any expected delays.

- Block time each day for walk-ins and emergencies. Fill these times no earlier than the evening before.

Documentation of appointment information is almost as critical as the progress note itself. Always document appointments using the following guidelines:

- Record missed or canceled appointments in the patient's chart.

- Do not erase, white out, or otherwise obliterate any appointment in the appointment book or computer schedule.

- Document any attempts to reach the patient to reschedule a missed appointment. If the patient's condition warrants, send a certified letter.

(See also Chapter 12, *Developing Policies and Procedures*, pp. 88–90.)

Billing and Collections

Many malpractice claims are initiated in response to the manner in which collection efforts are made. A written collection policy assures that all employees know what the policy is and how to handle each billing and collection situation. Consider addressing these issues in your policy:

- Patient education: Letting the patient know before his first appointment about your fee and payment requirements.

- A review procedure for circumstances that require special action.

- The patient's past payment history.

- The quality of care.

- The patient's satisfaction. If the patient balks at paying a bill, discuss it with him. Work out an agreeable payment arrangement, if possible.

- The cost of legal action versus how much money the patient owes. Obtain information from the appropriate small claims court in your area.

- Having the physician review every chart before initiating aggressive collection procedures.

- Understanding of patients' rights concerning privacy and the physician-patient relationship. (Do not send any medical information to a collection agency.)

- Awareness of Fair Debt Collection Act. (Periodically evaluate the collection agency's practices.)

(See also Chapter 13, *Billing and Reimbursement Protocols*, pp. 91-98.)

Environment

The patient develops a first impression of the kind of medical care he will receive when he views the practice surroundings. If the surroundings are pleasant, clean and convenient, patients will more likely view the physician as competent and providing quality care.

- To prevent patient injury, evaluate the facility to ensure easy access. All patient care areas should be checked, including the parking lot, to identify potential safety hazards.

- Provide comfortable office furnishings to allow the patient to feel at ease. Check furnishings periodically to assure that they are in good condition. Take steps to ensure cleanliness and good housekeeping. Messy or dirty offices create a negative impression. The effect on the patient's perception of quality is significant.

- Have furnishings that meet the needs of various patients. Soft and/or low seating is problematic for pregnant women, the elderly and the infirm.

- Keep the room at a comfortable temperature and provide plenty of lighting.

Medical Equipment

Patients are often injured because of faulty or improper use of equipment. The practice administrator should institute a policy of regular maintenance and use of all equipment.

- Train all employees on the proper use of equipment.

- Document the training, time, and place in each employee's personnel file.

- Calibrate all equipment as recommended by the manufacturer.

- Maintain a log of all equipment maintenance and service.

- Report any patient injury associated with a piece of equipment to your malpractice insurance carrier. Remove the equipment and all its collateral equipment from service.

- Avoid tampering with the equipment or sending it to the manufacturer for repair until you have notified the insurance company and they instruct you to do so.

- ***Do not document any assumptions about an equipment malfunction or improper usage in the medical record.***

Emergencies

All medical offices should have a written protocol for handling a medical emergency.

- Post emergency numbers such as ambulances, hospitals, poison control, etc., next to all telephones.

- Require all staff to stay current on cardiopulmonary resuscitation (CPR).

- If the office has emergency equipment and/or medications, train all staff to use such equipment and drugs. Not having this equipment on hand is better than to have untrained employees using it. There is often less liability in doing nothing than in doing something incorrectly.

- Conduct periodic emergency drills.

Confidentiality

Communication between the patient and physician is confidential. Patient confidentiality is critical to the patient/doctor relationship. Patients have filed many lawsuits due to breach of confidential information. It is the patient's right to decide what information the physician may reveal to others. This confidentiality privilege extends to all members of the health care team.

- All personal data, medical notes **and billing information** are confidential and may not be communicated to anyone without the patient's written consent.

- Do not discuss a patient's illness with any staff member who does not need to know.

- Do not discuss a patient's illness with family members or friends except in the presence of and with the consent of the patient.

- Loose talk that others overhear can be the basis for a defamation or invasion of privacy suit. Watch your voice volume; pay attention to who is nearby.

- Do a "confidentiality audit" of your office. Test to see how easy overhearing conversation is, particularly from the front office. If you need to, install some soundproofing.

- Avoid discussing a patient's medical care on a cellular phone with either the patient or anyone else. These conversations are sometimes picked up by police scanners and radios.

- Discuss confidentiality issues with all new employees. Make sure all staff members understand that violation of a patient's privacy is support for firing. Staff members should, at the time of hiring, sign a form pledging confidentiality of patient information; this form becomes a part of the personnel record.

Handling Patient Complaints

A patient shows dissatisfaction and intentions to sue long before the legal papers are served. A staff member may be the first to be aware of a patient complaint. No matter how incidental the complaint may seem, they must bring all complaints to the physician's attention.

- Institute a formal complaint policy in the office. Use an incident report form and a complaint log to track the occurrence and disposition of all patient complaints. Do not enter this information is in the patient's medical record.

- Notify the physician of the complaint on the day it is received.

- Respond to the complaint quickly and follow up with the patient.

Termination of the Patient/Physician Relationship

The inferred contract between a patient and a physician begins not when they make an appointment, but when examination or treatment begins. Once a physician-patient relationship has been established, the physician is not free to terminate the relationship at will without formal, written notification. The physician-patient relationship continues until it is ended by one of the following circumstances:

- The patient has no need of further care.
- The patient terminates the relationship.
- The physician formally terminates the relationship.

Failure to terminate may constitute patient abandonment and bring about fines or legal action if the patient is harmed by the abandonment.

There may be circumstances in which it is deemed necessary to terminate the physician-patient relationship. Perhaps the patient is noncompliant, and it is believed that continued treatment would increase the chances of a complication or poor outcome. Maybe the patient is rude or abusive, or maybe the physician and the patient just do not get along. Possibly the patient routinely fails to pay his bills. Any of those reasons and many others may be a reason to terminate a patient from your practice. If you do so, be sure to follow some specific guidelines to minimize the chance of being sued for abandonment.

A physician **cannot** refuse to give a patient an appointment because the patient has not paid the bill without first terminating the physician-patient relationship. This can be accomplished by sending the patient a **certified, return receipt letter**.

- First, put the notice in writing. The reason may or may not be stated.
  - If for noncompliance, say so clearly in the letter.
  - If for personality conflict, an unpaid bill, or for a reason not to be made public, avoid stating the reason in writing.
- Send the letter by certified mail, return receipt requested. Keep the receipt in the patient's file, along with a copy of the letter.

How much time that you are required to give a patient to seek alternative health care varies in each state. Contact your local medical society or attorney to find an answer. This termination process protects you from having to see the patient who fails to follow your suggested treatment plan.

The physician-patient relationship is the foundation of medical law. Upon it rests the legal rights and obligations of both patients and physicians. (See following *Sample Discharge Letter*.)

JAMES L. SMITH, M.D.
100 North Main Street
Anytown, U.S.A.

Telephone: (202) 555-1212

(Certified Mail-Return Receipt Requested)

Dear _____:

I find it necessary to inform you that I am withdrawing from further professional attendance upon you for the reason that you have persisted in refusing to follow my medical advice and treatment.

Since your condition requires medical attention, I suggest that you place yourself under the care of another physician without delay. If you so desire, I will be available to attend you for a reasonable time after you have received this letter, but in no event for more than thirty days.

This should give you ample time to select a physician of your choice from the many competent practitioners in this city. With your approval, I will make available to this physician your case history and information regarding the diagnosis and treatment that you have received from me.

Very truly yours,

_____ , M.D.

Rights of the Patient:

The patient has certain legal rights of which the physician and staff must be aware. These are as follows:

- The right to choose the physician from whom he or she wishes to receive treatment.

- The right to say whether medical treatment will begin and to set limits on the care provided.

- The right to know before the treatment begins what it will consist of, what effect it will have on the body, what are the inherent dangers, and what it will cost.

Consent to Treatment

Legal consequences for treating a patient without properly informed consent include charges of assault and battery and negligence. For emphasis, take note of the following:

- Treating a patient without permission is grounds for an assault and battery charge.

- Treating a patient with the patient's consent but failing to explain the inherent risks of a procedure could result in a charge of negligence.

Implied consent is reflected in the patient's actions such as having a prescription filled or accepting an injection.

Expressed consent is an oral or written acceptance of the treatment. Obtain the written form of expressed consent when the proposed treatment involves surgery, experimental drugs or procedures, or high-risk diagnostic or treatment procedures.

Informed Consent to Treatment

The fiduciary relationship between physician and patient is based on trust and confidence. The nature of this relationship obligates the physician to act for the benefit of the patient. Contained in this obligation is the physician's duty to voluntarily inform the patient of all relevant information concerning the treatment being offered including potential hazards and risks. This duty and legal principle that a mentally competent adult has control over his own body requires a physician to obtain the patient's informed consent before beginning medical treatment.

Informed consent will develop from the patient's understanding of the following factors:

- General nature of the treatment and consequences involved.

- Normal risks and hazards of inherent treatment.

- Side effects or complications known to occur.

- Alternative treatments.

Fraud and Abuse

Any medical practice treating Medicare patients must be aware of the strict fraud and abuse rules governing Medicare billing. The Office of Inspector General (OIG) is responsible for identifying and eliminating fraud and abuse. The OIG carries out this mission through a nationwide network of audits, investigations, and inspections of physicians' offices.

The most common inspection by the OIG is the Medicare audit. They conduct these audits to identify inconsistencies in billing, coverage, and payment of bills for particular services.

The HCFA defines Medicare fraud as "knowingly and willfully making or causing a false statement or representation of a material fact made in application for a Medicare benefit of payment." Fraud occurs when a physician knowingly bills Medicare for a service he did not render or when the physician overstates or exaggerates a particular service.

Some examples of Medicare fraud are as follows:

- An indication that there may be deliberate application of duplicate reimbursement.

- Any false representation with respect to the nature of charges for services rendered.

- A claim for uncovered services billed as services that are covered.

- A claim involving collusion between the physician and recipient resulting in higher costs or charges.

Medicare abuse refers to activities that may directly or indirectly cause financial losses to the Medicare program or the beneficiary. Abuse generally occurs when the physician operates in a manner inconsistent with accepted business and medical practices.

The most common types of abuse are:

- The overuse of medical services (e.g., repeated lab testing when results are normal, etc.)

- Up coding and overuse of office visits

- Waiving copayments. Physicians are required to collect the 20 percent Medicare copayment from the Medicare patient. Routinely waiving the copayment, unless in very unusual cases such as extreme financial hardship, is considered a fraudulent activity.

The Medical Record

A well documented, legible, structured medical record is the physician's first line of defense if there is a malpractice suit. The medical record is a form of communication among health care professionals about the patient's condition. This documentation identifies the patient, supports the diagnosis, justifies the treatment and documents the results of treatment.

The medical record is confidential. The information is private, should remain secure and not made public. While the record belongs to the physician, the information belongs to the patient.

Authorization to Release Records

Sole authority to release information from his medical record belongs to the patient. The office should be prepared with a printed release form that the patient signs to release the medical record to a third party. The release form need not be complicated or full of legal language.

As a word of caution, HIV/AIDS information is **not** included in a standard release form. The release form must **specifically** state that the release includes this information.

Any mention of HIV/AIDS testing or treatment is extremely sensitive and should be maintained in a separate part of the medical record. Some attorneys suggest it should be maintained in an envelope marked, *CONFIDENTIAL! DO NOT RELEASE.*

Records are the heart of systematic patient care. Excellent record keeping is one of the most effective tools in patient care and in preventing claims. Following are the key elements of a good medical record.

- **Uniform Records.** Medical records should be uniform within the practice. An excellent way to structure charts is to insert dividers for lab, x-ray, progress notes, etc., and to use a problem list. In this format, the record is organized for easy scanning by all health care professionals who subsequently use the chart.

- **Secure Pages.** Secure all pages of the record in chronological order with fasteners to prevent pages from being lost.

- **Organization.** Organize records for easy and accurate retrieval. Whatever system is used, it should be logical and clear to all staff members and physicians (e.g., active versus inactive patients, color coding for chronic problems or frequent diagnoses, etc.).

- **Timeliness.** Make all entries in the record, whether written or dictated, at the time of the patient contact. Include the date and the time of the exam or contact. The greater the time lapse between the exam and the entry, the less credible the medical record becomes.

- **Legible Records.** Records must be legible. Health care professionals with illegible handwriting should dictate their notes. This helps to avoid misinterpretations that result in improper treatment.

- **Dictated Records.** Dictated notes must be proofread and signed. The statement "dictated but not read" does not relieve the physician from responsibility for what was transcribed. At best, the statement alerts another health care professional that the note has not been proofed and may not be correct.

- **Accurate Records.** Recording all information in objective and concise terms is important. Never include extraneous information or subjective assessments of the patient, such as "this patient is a jerk." Include direct quotations from the patient. Reduce the essential information to the least possible number of words.

- **Corrections.** *Never* improperly or unlawfully alter a medical record. Do not obliterate an entry with a marker or white-out. If an error has been made, draw a single line through the inaccurate entry and enter the necessary correction. Date, time and initial the correction in the margin. Making an addendum to a medical record is also acceptable. It should be made after the last entry noting the current date and time, and both entries should be cross-referenced. A record that appears to have been altered implies that a cover-up has occurred.

- **Jousting.** Never criticize or make derogatory comments about another health care professional or organization to the patient or in the medical record. A negative comment can undermine a patient's confidence in the previous health care worker and contribute to or cause a decision to pursue a legal claim regardless of causation and/or who was responsible.

- **Patient Telephone Calls.** Document all patient telephone calls in the medical record. When speaking to a patient while you are away from the office, and the medical record is not available, record notes on a call pad regarding any prescriptions or medical advice given over the telephone. You can present the sheet for entry into the chart when you return to the office.

- **Conversations.** Address and document all patient/family worries or concerns in the patient record. Record the source of the information, if other than the patient.

- **Important Instructions.** Always document important warnings and instructions given to the patient at the time of discharge. Documenting discharge instructions may help prove a noncompliance. Juries are less sympathetic toward noncompliant patients.

- **Informed Consent.** To reinforce the signed informed consent form, always document information disclosed during the informed consent process.

- **Potential Complications.** Document all possible complications that might occur. Failure to recognize a complication in time to prevent injury is a common basis for lawsuit. Proving negligence is difficult if the record shows prior awareness that a complication might occur.

Medical Records Documentation

A great deal of emphasis has been placed recently on the thorough documentation of patient encounters. Not only is documentation critical to reduce the possibility of malpractice, it is also a necessity in claiming proper reimbursement.

Many physicians have been unsuccessful in defending a malpractice suit due to incomplete or illegible medical records. Malpractice insurance carriers and risk management experts recommend the following loss prevention tips:

- Fasten all materials into the chart.

- Dictate progress notes and have them transcribed if possible.

- Clearly identify allergies on the chart.

- The patient's name should be on every page in the chart.

- The physician should initial every entry in the medical record.

- Financial data should not be kept in the chart.

An example of a medical record review sheet has been provided at the end of the chapter. Assuring that these guidelines are being met by periodically check 10 to 20 charts is prudent.

Documentation to Support Level of Service

Most Managed Care Organizations (MCOs) have definite guidelines for documenting patient encounters. Sometimes they conduct post payment audits in the physician's office to assure that the documentation on the patient's medical chart supports the service charged, and to assure that the physician took the proper steps to reach a satisfactory diagnosis. Medicare also conducts post payment audits and will usually request that the physician mail in photocopies of specific patient records. Both MCOs and Medicare will require the physician to repay any amount paid for a service that is not supported by proper documentation. These repayments can sometimes amount to thousands of dollars.

In order for the physician to avoid this kind of risk, it is best to set up the patient records in the start-up phase of the practice to make thorough documentation as convenient and efficient as possible. Existing charts (inherited from other practitioners) can be converted over time to a more formal organization of the information. Preprinted forms for progress notes, medication records, telephone calls and other reports are recommended.

Charting the Patient's Progress

Using a standard format to record the patient's visit will assure that every encounter includes all the components necessary for complete documentation. The American Academy of Family Practice recommends the S.O.A.P. format.

When utilizing the S.O.A.P. format, the physician records the patient encounter in the following manner:

S = Subjective findings
O = Objective findings
A = Assessment of problem/complaint
P = Plan of treatment

This format is easily followed by any health care provider and should be complete if the record is ever subpoenaed in a legal case.

Organizing the Patient File

Having every patient's chart organized in the same manner is a time saver. It takes less time to locate a specific report or item the physician needs to properly treat the patient.

Below is an example of how a patient's chart might be organized for greater efficiency.

Chart Map

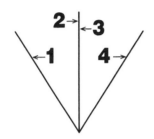

Side view of Chart with one flap

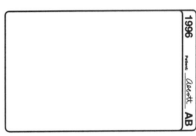

Front view of Chart

Section 1

Lab Reports
XRay Reports
EKG Reports

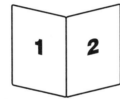

Section 2

Progress Notes
Including Telephone Messages

Physicals

Section 3

Demographics
Insurance Information
Insurance/Correspondence
Divider
Correspondence

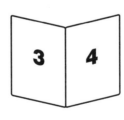

Section 4

Hospital/Consults

Medical Records Checklist Form

MEDICAL RECORDS CHECKLIST	Yes	No	N/A
Patient name on all pages			
All pages secured with fasteners			
Forms organized with tabs for easy access			
Organized chronologically			
Legible entries			
Missed appointments documented			
Telephone message documented			
Allergies uniformly documented			
Entries dated, timed and initialed			
Dictation proofread and initialed			
Only standard abbreviations used			
Diagnostic reports initialed prior to filing			
Reason for visit documented			
Clinical findings (positive/negative) documented			
Treatment plan documented			
Entries are objective			
Patient instructions documented			
Patient education materials given/documented			
Medication List			
1. current			
2. prescriptions			
3. refills			
4. allergies			
Informed consent on chart			
Referral letters on chart			
Consultation reports on chart			
Problem list kept current			

CHAPTER 15

Marketing

Developing Marketing Strategies

A rapidly changing health care environment is constantly challenging physicians to adopt strategies to attract new patients and maintain the loyalties of existing patients. Since the term "marketing" contains some negative connotations for physicians, think of these strategies as "enhancing" the practice. Whatever your description, these actions are a vital part of your success.

The strategies you employ to attract new patients are generally very tangible, such as yellow pages or newspaper advertisements. These are called external marketing strategies. Internal strategies are directed toward retaining the patient base and increasing loyalty through subliminal activities. The physician and staff accomplish these through friendliness and efficiency, expressed by communication and concern. This chapter will provide some suggestions on both internal and external marketing strategies.

The Marketing Budget

As you establish the first year's operational budget for your practice, include a specific amount for marketing expenses. Establishing a marketing budget is an extremely important step in the development of your promotional efforts. There are many ways to advance your practice, and every method has its costs. Do not consider these expenditures as optional; they are as vital to your success as having the proper equipment. If you do not expend the necessary time and money, you may suffer the consequences in loss of patients to your competition.

Obtain quotes on the development and printing of a practice brochure, appointment and business cards, letterhead, and other stationery, and educational materials. Factor these costs into your first year budget. Include the costs of any other marketing expense you might have such as your newspaper announcement and your yellow pages advertisement.

The Marketing Plan

Just as you have planned for the furniture and equipment needs in starting your practice, you will want to establish a marketing plan. The plan need not be complicated nor formal, but it is imperative that you commit it to paper. Share your plan with your staff. They will become an integral part of your marketing efforts.

Four months before opening:

Check sources such as *The Welcome Wagon* and groups that present information to new residents. Supply handout items for their distribution.

Set up a system to track how patients are referred to the practice. One method is to use a referral log, a simple grid that lists the various sources of referral. Referrals come from various sources, e.g., the newspaper, yellow pages, hearing a presentation you made to a civic group, from another physician or patient, etc. Always ask patients the name of the patient, physician or other individual that referred them to you. Send a note to that person saying, "Thank you for the referral."

Attend meetings and join civic groups that will enhance your presence in the community, such as the Rotary Club or the Civitans. If you have children in the local school system, joining the Parent-Teachers Association is fitting. Offer to speak to these organizations on medical topics. Tell the Medical Staff Secretary at your hospital(s) that you are available for public speaking engagements.

Check with local hospitals to see if these institutions have planned Health Fairs or Health Screenings in the future. Offer to participate.

Three months before opening:

Now is the time to develop your practice brochure. An attractive, well-prepared brochure provides your patients with all the information they need about your practice. Include a short paragraph about yourself, your specialty, and your education. A photograph adds a good touch. If your budget does not permit you to have a professionally prepared brochure, use a word processor and laser printer to print this information about your practice. An outline for a practice brochure is provided at the end of this chapter.

Two months before opening:

Design and order announcement cards to send to local physicians and other health care professionals. These announcements should show your name, specialty, address and telephone number; mail at least two weeks before you open.

Order stationery and appointment cards with your letterhead and your logo if you have developed one. Order only small amounts to begin. You may want to make changes later.

One month before opening:

Order patient education materials for the practice. Use a rubber stamp to imprint your name and address on the front of every piece of educational information you hand out or place in the waiting room. This information may find its way to another potential patient.

Visit the hospital(s) where you will be on staff. Introduce yourself to the department heads and nursing staff.

If you are providing treatment for work injuries, rehabilitation, or other occupationally related services, visit the employers in the area; introduce yourself and the services you provide. Take copies of your practice brochure and your business cards. Meet with the person responsible for Workers' Compensation injuries or treatment, and the benefits coordinator.

Two weeks before opening day:

Draft a newspaper advertisement and submit it to the local newspaper(s). The advertisement should give your name, address, and telephone number. It should define and briefly describe your specialty and the services you offer. Also, indicate your hours of operation.

Meet with your staff to share your marketing plan and ask for ideas. Patients who call for an appointment will want to know a little about you. Give each employee a copy of your Curriculum Vitae and outline your specialty training. Tell them about yourself so they can discuss your credentials with potential patients. Explaining to your staff the types of services provided by your specialty is also helpful. Keep in mind that your staff is "marketing" your services to patients.

Conduct office staff training on telephone communications to patients and referring physicians. If you receive a referral from a physician you have not previously met, it is a good idea to speak to that physician yourself. Put these protocols in writing and make them a part of your Policies and Procedures Manual. Tell your staff how much time you need for specific types of appointments. Allow extra time for any first visit; you will be building relationships during this time.

Practice Building Guidelines for the Future

With any marketing effort you enter, developing guidelines is important. Clarify your thoughts and plans on paper and follow these suggestions:

- *Define your objectives.* Define these for the short term (less than one year), then define them for the long term (more than one year). Express them in a quantifiable and trackable way. Otherwise, you never know whether you are succeeding or failing.

- *Caution!* Practically all professionals automatically say, "I'd like to double my practice." It is not as simple as that. Determine how much you are willing to spend to achieve that goal. To play conservatively, figure that your budget must amount to 20 to 33 percent of your targeted increase in income to generate an equally conservative 333 to 500 percent return on investment.

  Remember cash flow. Many strategies call for 50 to 75 percent of the marketing budget to be spent in the first 25 percent of the time. This usually means that the first large sum of cash needs to be in the bank at the start of the program, so it cannot come out of unexpected cash flow.

- *Identify your target groups.* Define the groups you are trying to reach. Describe your target populations by the chief characteristics of age, sex, location, educational level, income, ethnicity/religion, blue collar workers versus white collar workers, and lifestyle. Choose only those factors that are most important, usually income, education, sex, age, and location. If you target business, describe it by industry, industry position, yearly sales, number of employees, and location.

  Create a different, one-page marketing plan for each target, for example, other practitioners from whom to generate referrals, senior citizens, blue-collar workers, 18- to 34-year-old females, and so on. Then rank those groups, targeting the easiest first.

- *Define what the target groups want.* What are the characteristics most important to the target group in selecting a physician in your field? Is it experience, hours, location, price?

- *Define who you are.* What are your strengths? Weaknesses? What is different or special about you concerning your education, expertise, years of experience, credentials? What do you offer in location, hours, pricing, equipment?

- *Analyze your main competitors.* Analyze just the ones with whom you compete in your service area. Do not ignore the indirect competitors outside your profession to whom prospects could turn as a substitute, such as chiropractors, podiatrists, or psychologists. Chart each competitor's strengths and weaknesses.

- *How to compete.* How do you rate against those main competitors? Where can you best compete? List primary points. Then secondary points. Can you service your targets well, or are you going too far outside your area of expertise? Are you trying to draw from too great a distance?

  Assume you have good, solid experience, but that one of your competitors has more. If that competitor does not promote experience and you do, you will have the reputation for experience with the public. The same is true for any other advantage.

- *Determine your budget.* How much can you afford now? Reconcile your budget with your goals.

- *Choose your strategy.* Should it be internal promotion? Yellow pages? Newspapers? Public relations? Seminars? Is this strategy the most effective one? Weigh the pros and cons of various vehicles against each other.

- *Choose your timing.* List events, both external and internal, that will affect your campaign over the period you have specified. Choose the time of year, which months, and what week to take action. If your practice has seasonal peaks, promote heavily as you enter your busier periods, not during you practice lows. Your dollars and efforts must work a lot harder in low periods when prospects are not already looking for your services.

- *Plan your execution.* Assign responsibilities. Set deadlines for all steps on a master time line.

Building Patient Satisfaction

In a pure fee-for-service market, a patient's dissatisfaction with a physician generally amounts to the loss of that one patient and possibly the loss of another family member. In a market dominated by managed care organizations, patient dissatisfaction can result in the loss of an entire patient population.

Managed Care Organizations gather a tremendous amount of data from their enrollees and use this information as a component in "grading" the plan's physicians. If a physician fails to make the grade, they may drop him from the plan.

Be proactive in your attempts to increase patient satisfaction. After your practice has been established about six months, conduct a patient satisfaction survey. Survey at least one hundred patients or, if possible, every patient. You will gain invaluable opinions about your practice, your staff and about your own success up to this point. Take your patients' suggestions seriously. Carry out any changes that will increase patient satisfaction.

A sample survey is provided later in the chapter.

Practice Services and Amenities

Marketing can be as simple as making every patient feel comfortable and appreciated. Differentiate your practice from others by providing a personal touch to patient relationships. Follow these guidelines as a part of your approach to patient service:

- Assign someone in your office the responsibility of managing the practice's relationships with its most important customers.

- Send a welcome letter to a patient after they have made the initial appointment. Thank the patient and enclose a practice brochure.

- Acknowledge patients immediately upon arrival.

- Always address a patient by name. Be very sensitive to the patient's feelings in deciding whether to use formal or informal terms of address.

- Explain all lengthy delays, and make sure that patients are given the opportunity to reschedule if they so desire. The physician(s) should be encouraged to be punctual and attentive to the appointment schedule. Remember, the patient's time is valuable, too!

- Let disabled or elderly patients know that by prearrangement they can be met at their cars and escorted into the office. Have a wheelchair available.

- Provide educational materials; they usually result in patients who are more able and willing to assume responsibility in assisting you in the healing process. Many forms are available commercially, or you can write your own educational materials, produce your own video or audio cassettes, establish a lending library, etc.

- Ask about the patient's family. Some physicians jot down personal notes about each patient and keep them in the patient's chart. A few physicians even have photographs taken of each patient and attach them to charts to refresh the physician's memory.

- Spend adequate time with each patient. Surveys show that patient satisfaction directly correlates with how much time the physician spends with the patient.

- Create a pleasant reception area:
  - provide a living room effect
  - decorate tastefully
  - use table lamps rather than fluorescent lighting
  - display arrangements of fresh cut flowers
  - provide educational videos on interesting health topics
  - provide tasteful distractions such as an aquarium, art objects, wall hangings
  - play soothing, easy-listening music
  - offer patients something to do, e.g., puzzles, books, crossword puzzles, current magazines.

Standards of Patient Service for Medical Staff

Each member of your staff should render services to patients with the highest professional standards. The following guidelines serve as effective reminders of how best to treat patients.

- Acknowledge patients promptly and courteously with eye contact and a pleasant expression and tone of voice.

- When talking with patients and/or other employees, use words that express respect, patience, and understanding.

- Care for people with kindness and gentleness, rather than with cold professionalism.

- Address adult patients by their proper title and last name, unless the patient requests otherwise.

- Display visible identification and introduce yourself by name and title when first meeting a patient.

- Answer the telephone quickly and courteously, identify yourself by name. Provide callers the opportunity to respond to a request to be placed on hold, and explain to them if their call is being transferred.

- Be sensitive to reducing noise levels near patient care areas.

- Respect patient privacy by knocking before entering the room if the door is closed, and by refraining from discussing one patient in front of another.

- Protect the confidentiality of patients, coworkers and others who use the facilities.

- Make certain that patient modesty is respected always.

- Be attentive to patients and their families who are kept waiting in waiting areas or treatment rooms for extended periods.

- Consider the effect of what you say and do in the presence of patients. Refrain from conducting personal (not work-related) conversations in front of patients.

- Refrain from discussing other employees, organizational policies, problems or medical care in public areas.

- Maintain and use medical equipment and facilities appropriately and cost-effectively.

Yellow Pages Advertising

A well-designed Yellow Pages advertisement can work for you 24 hours a day, 365 days a year. Statistics suggest that practices attract 5 to 10 percent of their new patients through Yellow Pages advertising. They are also useful for attracting patients who have not been to your practice for some time.

Before placing your ad, evaluate what your colleagues are doing. Then look through the Yellow Pages from another community and compare styles, design, size and text. What makes the ad stand out from the rest? Which ads are you attracted to?

The goal is to make your ad unique and grab the attention of the shopper. Achieving this without discrediting your practice with a cluttered distasteful ad is very important. A simple, clean, and professionally designed 2" x 3" ad can be very effective. The following checklist will help you create an effective, powerful and attractive ad.

- Are your name, specialty and phone number the most prominent elements in your ad?

- Have you included the name of the practice with the name(s) of the physician(s) in the practice?

- Have you included any special qualifications such as board certification?

- Do you want to mention area locators such as cross streets or building names, with listing your office address?

- If you offer extended hours, have you listed them?

- If you offer any special services, have you included them?

- If you have a logo or slogan, have you included them in your ad?

- Have you reviewed the ad sizes of your competition to determine the ad size you need for your ad to stand out?

- Have you considered using boldface type to call attention to your ad?

- Have you chosen a typeface that corresponds to the character of your practice?

- Does the ad reflect the image you want to project for your practice?

Creating a Medical Practice Brochure

A practice brochure creates many marketing opportunities. It creates an image of your practice to current and prospective patients and referral sources. Your brochure provides information about your services, office policies, and practice philosophy. It also saves staff time by addressing repetitive questions, such as where you have hospital privileges or how to bill their insurance. The brochure will serve as a compact reference about your practice.

How to Create a Brochure

The best resources for creating a brochure are your colleagues and other professional businesses. To obtain ideas, collect samples of attractive brochures. A typical brochure has six to eight panels of information and is 3-1/2" x 8-1/2". Write your own copy or hire a professional to help you. The goal of the brochure is to clarify your practice policies. Whoever writes it should use language that is clear, concise and easy to understand.

Brochure Contents

The practice brochure should contain the following information:

Introduction to the Practice. Begin by including the name, address and telephone number of the practice. Provide a brief history of the practice and state the patient care and philosophy.

Professional Profile of the Physician(s). Introduce each physician in the practice and include detail on training, board certification, areas of special interest and personal information. For example, "Dr. Doe is married and has two lovely children," or "Dr. Smith enjoys working in under-served countries one month each year." Include a picture of each physician to help patients with name and face recognition.

Explanation of Specialty. Quite frequently, physicians and their staffs are not aware that patients do not know or understand a physician's specialty and the part of the anatomy to which it pertains. They assume that once a patient gets as far as the reception room, the patient has a clear and thorough understanding of why he is there. To educate the patient about the practice, include a description, in simple terms, of the practice specialty and the special services and procedures you provide. The more informed a patient is before the visit, the more confidence the patient can have in the care received.

Office Policies. One primary objective of a practice brochure is to educate and inform patients about practice policies. It serves as a reference and reminder to established patients and provides guidelines and standards for new patients before incurring services.

Key areas to highlight include:

Office Hours. This is especially critical if your appointment times are beyond the "typical" practice hours, i.e., evening or Saturday hours. Stating office hours will also reduce after-hours calls to the answering service and consequently reduce overhead expenses.

How to Schedule and Cancel Appointments. If you ask that your patients use a different telephone number for scheduling appointments, publicize it. If you have many "no-show" patients, it is very important to establish and state the policy that will discourage this abuse and encourage compliance. Charging $25 for a no-show or a late cancellation is customary for practices (within 24 hours of scheduled appointment). If a patient abuses either policy three times, he should receive a letter discharging him from care within a reasonable period (i.e., 30 days). To protect the practice, send the letter via certified mail, return receipt requested.

Hospital Affiliations. The insurance industry may influence a patient's selection of both a hospital and a physician. Therefore, including your hospital affiliations in the practice brochure is important.

Financial Policies. Generally, the most frequently asked questions pertain to the practice's financial policies. Document these policies in the brochure to inform patients about their financial responsibility.

Include the forms of accepted payment, i.e., cash, check, credit card. Most practices follow the policy that they expect payment when they render services unless the patient makes other arrangements. This policy should be stated. Identify the insurance plans in which you participate, e.g., IPA, PPO, HMO. Also state if you do or do not accept Medicare assignment. Include billing information, such as when the patient should expect to receive a statement, after what period an account will be placed in collection, etc. Be sure to include the telephone number to call regarding billing question.

Special Services. Health care consumers will look for practices that offer "one-stop-shopping." List all services the practice offers, such as laboratory and radiology services. Also list special procedures or testing that are offered, e.g., infertility tests, nutrition counseling, pain management, etc.

Telephone Calls. If your practice has an established office policy regarding prescription refills, print it in the brochure. Patients need to know how to handle routine prescription refills. Informing them of your policy makes the office more efficient and responsive to the patient's request.

Notifying patients that an answering service will respond to calls after normal office hours is important. Patients appreciate knowing a voice is always on the other end of the line, and that the physician will get their message. You may consider printing the answering service telephone number for the rare occasion the office forgets to sign off to the service after hours. Printing the physician's pager number is not advisable.

Map of Office Location. Including a map of your office location is as important as printing the name and telephone number of the practice. The map should include landmarks, such as a hospital, a lake, a park or something with which the patient may be familiar. If the office is close to the hospital, it adds a competitive marketing edge. It is to your benefit to include this information.

Patient Satisfaction Survey

		YES	NO
1.	Do you feel you understand the specialty of our practice?	❏	❏
2.	Do you believe you are aware of all the services we offer?	❏	❏
3.	Is the location of our office convenient?	❏	❏
4.	Do you find our waiting room comfortable?	❏	❏
5.	Do you feel relaxed in the waiting room?	❏	❏
6.	Are our parking facilities adequate?	❏	❏
7.	Do you have to pay to park when you come to see us?	❏	❏
8.	If yes, is this a hindrance to receiving your care here?	❏	❏
9.	Do you have to pay to park when you see other practitioners?	❏	❏
10.	What change would you make in the physician aspects of our office?	❏	❏
11.	Do you find our front office personnel (secretary, receptionist, etc.) friendly?	❏	❏
	Courteous?	❏	❏
12.	Do you find our business personnel (practice manager, bookkeeper, etc.) friendly?	❏	❏
	Courteous?	❏	❏
13.	Are your phone calls handled in a prompt, courteous, manner?	❏	❏
14.	Are you receiving adequate help with your insurance?	❏	❏
15.	Have you received a copy of our business policies?	❏	❏
16.	Have our payment and billing policies been explained to your satisfaction?	❏	❏
17.	Do you find our nurses friendly?	❏	❏
	Courteous?	❏	❏
18.	Do you feel our nurses are sympathetic to your illness?	❏	❏
19.	Do you find the doctor(s) friendly?	❏	❏
	Courteous?	❏	❏
20.	Do you feel the doctor is interested in you as a person?	❏	❏
21.	Does the doctor spend enough time with you?	❏	❏
22.	Is your wait too long in the reception area before you see the doctor?	❏	❏

		YES	NO
23.	Do you have to wait too long in the examination room before you see the doctor?	❏	❏
24.	Is our answering service prompt and courteous?	❏	❏
25.	Do our doctors promptly return your calls?	❏	❏
26.	Are your phone calls to the doctors during the day?	❏	❏
27.	Do you mind if the nurses respond to some of your calls?	❏	❏
28.	Are you satisfied with the hospital we use?	❏	❏
29.	Is this hospital convenient for you and your family?	❏	❏
30.	Do you feel that our fees are high?	❏	❏
	Average?	❏	❏

31. Have you used other health services (such as an emergency clinic) because you felt it would be less expensive? If yes, which one(s)?

_____

		YES	NO
32.	Do you have trouble getting an appointment when you would like?	❏	❏
33.	Are our secretaries helpful in finding appointments that meet your needs?	❏	❏
34.	Are our office hours convenient for you?	❏	❏

If not, how could we better serve you? _____

_____

		YES	NO
35.	Would you like more educational information from us?	❏	❏
36.	If we have audiovisual tapes available about your medical problem, would you use them?	❏	❏
37.	Would you want to receive a health newsletter from us periodically?	❏	❏

38. How were you referred to this practice?

❏ Other patients ❏ Friends ❏ Yellow Pages ❏ Medical society ❏ Another doctor

❏ Our reputation ❏ Other:_____

39.	Are you satisfied enough with the care we provide to refer other people to us?	❏	❏

Bibliography

Buster, Victoria. "Taking Care of Business." *Unique Opportunities,* November/December, 1994, Volume 4, Number 6, pp. 17-18.

Meyer, William G., III. "Accounting Essentials." *Unique Opportunities,* November/December, 1994, Volume 4, Number 6, pp. 36-43.

Pontius, C. Anne. "CDC Announces Seven New CLIA Tests Waived." *MGMA Update,* May, 1996, Volume 35, Number 5, p. 5.

PRACTICE SUCCESS! Norcross, GA: Coker Publishing, LLC., 1994.

Starting to Practice Smart. Chicago, IL: American Medical Association Financing & Practice Services, Inc., 1993.

Tinsley, Reed, C.P.A. "Your Guide to Starting a Practice." *Unique Opportunities,* November/December, 1994, Volume 4, Number 6, pp. 21-35.

Zicconi, John. "Beat the Financial Blues." *Unique Opportunities,* November/December, 1994, Volume 4, Number 6, pp. 44-51.

Index

S

T, U, V

W, X, Y, Z